Cardiovascular Emergencies

Editors

JEREMY G. BERBERIAN
LEEN ALBLAIHED

EMERGENCY MEDICINE CLINICS OF NORTH AMERICA

www.emed.theclinics.com

Consulting Editor
AMAL MATTU

November 2022 • Volume 40 • Number 4

ELSEVIER

1600 John F. Kennedy Boulevard • Suite 1800 • Philadelphia, Pennsylvania, 19103-2899

http://www.theclinics.com

EMERGENCY MEDICINE CLINICS OF NORTH AMERICA Volume 40, Number 4
November 2022 ISSN 0733-8627, ISBN-13: 978-0-323-98701-1

Editor: Joanna Collett
Developmental Editor: Axell Ivan Jade Purificacion

Emergency Medicine Clinics of North America (ISSN 0733-8627) is published quarterly by Elsevier Inc., 360 Park Avenue South, New York, NY, 10010-1710. Months of issue are February, May, August, and November. Business and Editorial Offices: 1600 John F. Kennedy Boulevard, Suite 1800, Philadelphia, PA 19103-2899. Customer Service Office: 6277 Sea Harbor Drive, Orlando, FL 32887-4800. Periodicals postage paid at New York, NY, and additional mailing offices. Subscription prices are $100.00 per year (US students), $370.00 per year (US individuals), $963.00 per year (US institutions), $220.00 per year (international students), $476.00 per year (international individuals), $1002.00 per year (international institutions), $100.00 per year (Canadian students), $436.00 per year (Canadian individuals), and $1002.00 per year (Canadian institutions). International air speed delivery is included in all *Clinics'* subscription prices. All prices are subject to change without notice. **POSTMASTER:** Send address changes to *Emergency Medicine Clinics of North America*, Elsevier Periodicals Customer Service, 11830 Westline Industrial Drive, St. Louis, MO 63146. Customer Service (orders, claims, online, change of address): Elsevier Periodicals **Customer Service, 11830 Westline Industrial Drive, St. Louis, MO 63146. Tel: 1-800-654-2452 (U.S. and Canada); 314-453-7041 (outside U.S. and Canada). Fax: 314-453-5170. E-mail: journalscustomerservice-usa@elsevier.com (for print support); journalsonlinesupport-usa@elsevier.com (for online support).**

Reprints. For copies of 100 or more of articles in this publication, please contact the Commercial Reprints Department, Elsevier Inc., 360 Park Avenue South, New York, NY 10010-1710. Tel.: 212-633-3874; Fax: 212-633-3820; E-mail: reprints@elsevier.com.

Emergency Medicine Clinics of North America is covered in *MEDLINE/PubMed (Index Medicus), Current Contents/Clinical Medicine, EMBASE/Excerpta Medica, BIOSIS, SciSearch, CINAHL, ISI/BIOMED,* and *Research Alert.*

Contributors

CONSULTING EDITOR

AMAL MATTU, MD, FAAEM, FACEP
Professor and Vice Chair of Academic Affairs, Department of Emergency Medicine, University of Maryland School of Medicine, Baltimore, Maryland, USA

EDITORS

JEREMY G. BERBERIAN, MD
Associate Director of Emergency Medicine Residency Education, Assistant Professor, Department of Emergency Medicine, ChristianaCare, Newark, Delaware, USA

LEEN ALBLAIHED, MBBS, MHA
Assistant Professor, Department of Emergency Medicine, University of Maryland School of Medicine, Baltimore, Maryland, USA

AUTHORS

MOHAMMED ALAGEEL, MBBS
Assistant Professor, Department of Emergency Medicine, King Saud University, Riyadh, Saudi Arabia; Clinical Instructor, Department of Emergency Medicine, University of British Columbia, Vancouver, British Columbia, Canada

LEEN ALBLAIHED, MBBS, MHA
Assistant Professor, Department of Emergency Medicine, University of Maryland School of Medicine, Baltimore, Maryland, USA

TAREQ AL-SALAMAH, MBBS, MPH
Assistant Professor, Adjunct Clinical Instructor, Department of Emergency Medicine, King Saud University, Riyadh, Saudi Arabia; Clinical Instructor, Department of Emergency Medicine, University of Maryland School of Medicine, Baltimore, Maryland, USA

JOEL ATWOOD, MD
Department of Emergency Medicine, York, Pennsylvania, USA

JEREMY G. BERBERIAN, MD
Associate Director of Emergency Medicine Residency Education, Assistant Professor, Department of Emergency Medicine, ChristianaCare, Newark, Delaware, USA

MICHAEL C. BOND, MD, FACEP, FAAEM
Professor, Department of Emergency Medicine, University of Maryland School of Medicine, Baltimore, Maryland, USA

ROBERT M. BROWN, MD
Assistant Professor, Department of Emergency Medicine, Virginia Tech Carilion School of Medicine, Roanoke, Virginia, USA

BRYAN D. HAYES, PharmD
Department of Pharmacy, Massachusetts General Hospital, Department of Emergency Medicine, Division of Medical Toxicology, Harvard Medical School, Boston, Massachusetts, USA

TYLER THOMAS HEMPEL, MD
Department of Emergency Medicine, Clerkship Director, UPMC Harrisburg, Harrisburg, Pennsylvania, USA

AKILESH HONASOGE, MD
Rush University, Chicago, Illinois, USA

KAMI M. HU, MD, FAAEM, FACEP
Departments of Emergency and Internal Medicine, University of Maryland School of Medicine, Baltimore, Maryland, USA

CHRISTINE S. JI, PharmD
Department of Pharmacy, Massachusetts General Hospital, Boston, Massachusetts, USA

JENNIFER L. KOEHL, PharmD
Department of Pharmacy, Massachusetts General Hospital, Boston, Massachusetts, USA

DANIEL L. KREIDER, MD
Emergency Physician, Advanced Emergency Medicine, Ultrasonography Fellowship Director, Department of Emergency Medicine, Wellspan York Hospital, York, Pennsylvania, USA

PHILLIP D. MAGIDSON, MD, MPH
Assistant Professor, Department of Emergency Medicine, Division of Geriatric Medicine and Gerontology, Johns Hopkins School of Medicine, Baltimore, Maryland, USA

JESSICA M. MASON, PharmD
Department of Pharmacy, Massachusetts General Hospital, Boston, Massachusetts, USA

MICHAEL E. O'BRIEN, PharmD
Department of Pharmacy, Massachusetts General Hospital, Boston, Massachusetts, USA

JOBIN PHILIP, MD
Department of Emergency Medicine, University of Maryland Medical Center, Baltimore, Maryland, USA

MAHESH POLAVARAPU, MD, FAAEM
Assistant Professor, Department of Emergency Medicine, Columbia University Irving Medical Center, New York, New York, USA

JOHN RIGGINS Jr, MD
Clinical Instructor, Department of Emergency Medicine, Columbia University Irving Medical Center, New York, New York, USA

WILLIAM BRANDON WHITE, DO
Department of Emergency Medicine, Emergency Medicine and Internal Medicine Chief Resident, ChristianaCare, Newark, Delaware, USA

AMY WYATT, DO
Department of Emergency Medicine, Associate Program Director, UPMC Harrisburg, Harrisburg, Pennsylvania, USA

Contents

Foreword: Cardiovascular Emergencies   **xiii**

Amal Mattu

Preface: Heart of the Matter   **xv**

Jeremy G. Berberian and Leen Alblaihed

Acute Coronary Syndrome in Women   **629**

Robert M. Brown

> Acute coronary syndrome is pathologically distinct in women and requires an appreciation of the specific risk factors, presenting symptoms, laboratory findings, and imaging results to treat correctly. Persistent disparities in mortality between men and women may be the result of failure to recognize and intervene, especially in the case of women aged less than 55 years. Protocols which establish criteria for activating the cardiac catheterization laboratory and which empower emergency department physicians to do so without delay show signs of eliminating disparities, as does guideline-directed therapy at the time of discharge from the hospital.

The Aged Heart   **637**

Phillip D. Magidson

> As the US populations ages, emergency medicine providers will require increased understanding of and expertise in the care of older adults presenting to the emergency department. No more is this evident than within the domain of cardiovascular emergency care. Cardiovascular emergencies and complications related to an aging cardiovascular system are some of the most common reasons this patient populations presents for emergency evaluation. This article provides guidance on the nuances of evaluation and treatment associated with these diseases in the older adult population.

Hereditary Syndromes of Sudden Cardiac Death   **651**

Jeremy G. Berberian

> Sudden cardiac death (SCD) describes the unexpected natural death from a cardiac cause within a short time period, generally 1 hour or lesser from the onset of symptoms, often due to a cardiac dysrhythmia. Overall, the most common cause of SCD is coronary artery disease but for patients aged younger than 35 years, the most common cause of SCD is a dysrhythmia in the setting of a structurally normal heart. This article will review the background, diagnosis, and management of the common hereditary channelopathies and cardiomyopathies associated with an increased risk of SCD in patients without ischemic heart disease.

The Ischemic Electrocardiogram   663

Daniel L. Kreider

> The electrocardiogram (EKG) is a useful diagnostic tool that allows clinicians to rapidly evaluate patients for acute coronary syndrome. With the high prevalence of heart disease in society, the EKG is crucial in the evaluation of chest pain and diagnosis of ischemia. Various guidelines provide criteria to aid in recognizing ischemia and help dictate patient management. Not all ischemic patterns requiring emergent management present within the classic definition of an STEMI. It is critical for clinicians to be able to accurately recognize these ischemic patterns to allow timely and appropriate cardiovascular care.

Pacemaker Malfunction–Review of Permanent Pacemakers and Malfunctions Encountered in the Emergency Department   679

William Brandon White and Jeremy G. Berberian

> Pacemaker malfunction refers to a failure of the pacemaker to perform the desired cardiac pacemaking function. These malfunctions can occur anywhere within the system from the pulse generator and leads to the electrode–myocardium interface. These failures of sensing, capture, and inadequate pacing can have severe hemodynamic consequences, so rapid identification of specific dysfunction is critical to intervention and stabilization. Emergency providers should be aware of pacemaker components, function, basic programming, and types of malfunctions to adequately assess, stabilize, and disposition patients.

Management of Acute Coronary Syndrome   693

Joel Atwood

> One of the most common complaints encountered in the emergency department is chest pain. In many evaluations, the leading diagnostic consideration is an acute coronary syndrome (ACS). ACS refers to a spectrum of coronary artery pathologies, including unstable angina, non-ST segment elevation myocardial infarction, and ST-segment elevation myocardial infarction. The distinction between subtypes of ACS guides acute diagnostic and management decisions. Failure to diagnose and manage ACS properly is a frequent cause of medico-legal litigation. In this article, we review the initial identification and critical management steps in patients presenting to the emergency department with ACS.

Medico-Legal Topics in Emergency Cardiology   707

John Riggins Jr. and Mahesh Polavarapu

> The workup and diagnosis of cardiovascular emergencies represent the present and future risk to emergency physicians. Eliciting and documenting key details of a cardiovascular complaint, as well as following established standards for accurate and timely diagnosis of emergencies, is central to the medico-legal aspects of cardiovascular emergencies. Key elements of documentation include history, physical exam, diagnostic workup, and medical decision making. Key elements of medical malpractice include the existence of a legal duty, breach of the legal duty,

causation, and presence of damages. All 4 legal elements must be present for medical malpractice to be proven in a court of law.

Narrow Complex Tachycardias   717

Tareq Al-Salamah, Mohammed AlAgeel, and Leen Alblaihed

Narrow-complex tachycardias are commonly seen on shift in the emergency department. Although a portion of patients present with hemodynamic instability because of arrhythmia, it is important to know that the tachycardia can be a result of an underlying condition. Rapid identification of the type and etiology of the arrhythmia is vital to directing appropriate management strategies and disposition decisions.

Wide Complex Tachycardias   733

Leen Alblaihed and Tareq Al-Salamah

Wide complex tachycardias (WCT) are frequently encountered in the emergency department. Causes of WCT vary from benign (eg, supraventricular with rate-related aberrancy) to life threatening (eg, atrial fibrillation with WPW, or ventricular tachycardia). It is imperative that emergency physicians are familiar with the clinical presentation, underlying causes, and electrocardiographic features of the different causes of WCT. Treatment of WCT depends on patient stability, regularity of the rhythm, and QRS morphology. When in doubt, monomorphic WCT should be presumed to be ventricular tachycardia and treated as such.

Emergency Department Evaluation and Management of Patients with Left Ventricular Assist Devices   755

Akilesh Honasoge and Kami M. Hu

With the increasing use of left ventricular assist devices (LVADs) as destination therapy in patients with severe left heart failure, emergency physicians are more likely to encounter patients with LVAD in their emergency department (ED). Emergency physicians should have a basic understanding of LVAD mechanics, a specific approach to LVAD patient evaluation, and awareness of the must-not-miss LVAD therapy complications and their management to optimize outcomes in this patient population.

Cardiovascular Pharmacology   771

Jessica M. Mason, Michael E. O'Brien, Jennifer L. Koehl, Christine S. Ji, and Bryan D. Hayes

Pharmacologic therapy is an integral component in the management of most cardiovascular emergencies. This article reviews the pharmacotherapy involved in the treatment of acute coronary syndromes, acute heart failure, and various arrhythmias. The focus will be to provide practical pearls that can be applied at the bedside in the Emergency Department.

Emergency Considerations of Infective Endocarditis   793

Jobin Philip and Michael C. Bond

Although still a rare bacterial infection of the endocardium of the heart, the incidence of infective endocarditis continues to increase with the increased use of intracardiac devices, indwelling lines, and surgical procedures being done on patients. The diagnosis of infective endocarditis remains challenging and requires a high level of suspicion to initiate the appropriate investigation and treatment. Serious complications can still occur despite optimal care, so it is helpful that these patients be managed by a team that includes infectious disease, cardiology, and cardiac surgeons.

High Sensitivity Troponins   809

Tyler Thomas Hempel and Amy Wyatt

High-sensitivity cardiac troponin (hs-cTn) assays are highly specific to cardiac tissue and can detect small amounts of myocardial injury rapidly. Hs-cTn assays are the recommended cardiac biomarkers in the major US and European guidelines. In the appropriate clinical context, these assays allow clinicians to rapidly rule out a non-ST-elevation myocardial infarction and decrease 30-day major adverse cardiac events. This can have significant downstream impacts on the percentage of patients discharged from the emergency department (ED), ED lengths of stay, cardiac testing, and hospitalizations. There are many proposed diagnostic protocols and experts recommend institutions implement a single validated protocol.

EMERGENCY MEDICINE CLINICS OF NORTH AMERICA

FORTHCOMING ISSUES

February 2023
Trauma Emergencies
Christopher M. Hicks and
Kimberly A. Boswell, *Editors*

May 2023
Updates in Obstetric and Gynecologic Emergencies
Sarah B. Dubbs and Brittany Guest, *Editors*

August 2023
Cardiac Arrest
William J. Brady and Amandeep Singh, *Editors*

RECENT ISSUES

August 2022
Respiratory and Airway Emergencies
Haney Mallemat and Terren Trott, *Editors*

May 2022
Toxicology Emergencies
Christopher P. Holstege and Joshua D. King, *Editors*

February 2022
Allergy, Inflammatory, and Autoimmune Disorders in Emergency Medicine
Gentry Wilkerson, Salvador J. Suau, *Editors*

SERIES OF RELATED INTEREST

Chest Medicine
https://www.chestmed.theclinics.com/
Critical Care Clinics
https://www.criticalcare.theclinics.com/

THE CLINICS ARE NOW AVAILABLE ONLINE!
Access your subscription at:
www.theclinics.com

FORTHCOMING ISSUES

February 2023
Trauma Emergencies
Christopher M. Hicks and
Elizabeth A. Beaulieu, Editors

May 2023
Updates in Obstetric and Gynecology
Emergencies
Sarah B. Dubbs and Brittany E. Davis, Editors

August 2023
Cardiac Arrest
William J. Brady and Amandeep Singh,
Editors

RECENT ISSUES

August 2022
Respiratory and Airway Emergencies
Haney Mallemat and Terren Trott, Editors

May 2022
Toxicology Emergencies
Christopher P. Holstege and Joshua D.
King, Editors

February 2022
Allergy, Inflammatory, and Autoimmune
Disorders Emergency Medicine
Gerald Wydro, Salvador J. Suau,
Editors

SERIES OF RELATED INTEREST

Pain Medicine
https://www.pmr.theclinics.com
Critical Care Clinics
https://www.criticalcare.theclinics.com

Foreword

Cardiovascular Emergencies

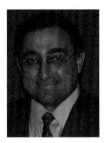

Amal Mattu, MD, FAAEM, FACEP
Consulting Editor

Emergency cardiac conditions are very common in the emergency department (ED). That statement should come as no surprise to any practitioner in emergency medicine (EM), but to highlight just how common these conditions are, I'd like to review the patients I saw during my shift in the ED: during my 8-hour shift, I cared for four patients presenting with chest pain; one patient presenting with acute heart failure; one patient presenting with syncope; one patient presenting with new-onset atrial fibrillation; and one patient presenting with concerns pertaining to his ventricular assist device. This group of patients constituted one-third of the new patients I evaluated during my shift, and I didn't feel like this was unusual for our ED.

Cardiac emergencies are not only common but also represent high-risk conditions. Cardiac conditions constitute the greatest cause of death in developed countries, and they also account for a significant percentage of money paid out in medical malpractice cases against emergency physicians in the United States. For these reasons, emergency physicians and any other acute care providers *must* commit themselves to staying up-to-date on advances in optimal care of patients presenting with emergency cardiac conditions.

In this issue of *Emergency Medicine Clinics of North America*, Guest Editors Drs Jeremy Berberian and Leen Alblaihed have assembled an outstanding group of authors to address many of the high-risk and cardiac conditions that we face in the specialty of EM. Articles address two groups of patients who are high risk for misdiagnosis of acute coronary syndrome: women and the elderly. Many key points in electrocardiography are addressed in articles on hereditary syndromes in sudden cardiac death, the ischemic electrocardiograms, pacemaker malfunction, and both narrow and wide complex tachycardias. In each of these articles, diagnosis as well as management is addressed. As ventricular assist devices become more common in our society, it is increasingly important for all acute care practitioners to understand these devices, and an excellent article is provided that addresses this often-confusing topic. Articles

Emerg Med Clin N Am 40 (2022) xiii–xiv
https://doi.org/10.1016/j.emc.2022.09.001
0733-8627/22/© 2022 Published by Elsevier Inc.

are also provided on acute coronary syndromes and troponins, endocarditis, and medical malpractice. Finally, a detailed review of cardiovascular pharmacology is provided.

This issue of *Emergency Medicine Clinics of North America* is an outstanding update to the knowledge base that most acute care practitioners have of emergency cardiology. I know that this entire issue will be incorporated into the reading curriculum for our EM residency, and I anticipate that these articles will advance the clinical care and competency of anyone involved in EM, from trainee to seasoned practitioner. The Guest Editors and authors are to be commended for providing this outstanding resource for our specialty.

Amal Mattu, MD, FAAEM, FACEP
Department of Emergency Medicine
University of Maryland School of Medicine
110 South Paca Street
6th Floor, Suite 200
Baltimore, MD 21201, USA

E-mail address:
amattu@som.umaryland.edu

Preface

Heart of the Matter

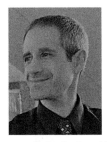   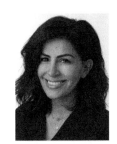

Jeremy G. Berberian, MD   Leen Alblaihed, MBBS, MHA
Editors

We are excited to share with you this issue of *Emergency Medicine Clinics of North America* covering cardiovascular emergencies. As with prior issues, choosing the topics was a challenging task. Our goal was to provide the reader with a diverse range of content, including underrepresented topics (ACS in women, cardiovascular considerations for geriatric patients), core content review (pacemaker abnormalities, narrow and wide complex tachydysrhythmias, endocarditis), updated core content (the ischemic ECG, hereditary syndromes of cardiac death, cardiovascular pharmacology, ACS management), and cutting-edge topics (high-sensitivity troponins, medicolegal topics in emergency cardiology).

We are grateful to all of the authors for their contributions to this issue. Their expertise in their respective topics is reflected in the concise yet thorough nature of each article. We are also grateful for the *Emergency Medicine Clinics of North America*

Emerg Med Clin N Am 40 (2022) xv–xvi
https://doi.org/10.1016/j.emc.2022.08.001
0733-8627/22/© 2022 Published by Elsevier Inc.

editorial staff for all their work in making this issue of Cardiovascular Emergencies. We hope you find this information useful in your clinical practice.

Jeremy G. Berberian, MD
Department of Emergency Medicine
ChristianaCare
4755 Ogletown Stanton Road
Newark, DE 19718, USA

Leen Alblaihed, MBBS, MHA
Department of Emergency Medicine
University of Maryland, School of Medicine
110 South Paca Street, Sixth Floor, Suite 200
Baltimore, MD 21201, USA

E-mail addresses:
jgberberian@gmail.com (J.G. Berberian)
lalblaihed@som.umaryland.edu (L. Alblaihed)

Acute Coronary Syndrome in Women

Robert M. Brown, MD*

KEYWORDS

- Women • ACS • CAD • SCAD • CMVD

KEY POINTS

- Acute coronary syndrome (ACS) encompasses acute thrombotic occlusion of coronary arteries as well as coronary microvascular dysfunction, coronary vasospasm, spontaneous coronary artery dissection, and Takotsubo cardiomyopathy.
- Presentations may be marked by symptoms such as fatigue, dyspnea, weakness, and pain in the jaw, neck, and upper back.
- High sensitivity troponins have different thresholds for ACS in men and women.
- Assessment with coronary angiography is appropriate with elevated troponin but assessment with coronary artery calcium score, optical coherence tomography, myocardial perfusion PET scanning, or intravascular ultrasound may be more appropriate otherwise.
- Protocolized and guideline-based care provided quickly to men and women eliminates sex disparities in mortality.

INTRODUCTION

Definition

Acute coronary syndrome (ACS) is the umbrella term for sudden myocardial ischemia or infarction resulting from diseases of the coronary circulation. ACS encompasses abrupt rupture of atherosclerotic plaque with thrombotic occlusion of a coronary artery as well as plaque erosion with endothelial dysfunction, microembolization, coronary vasospasm, toxicity from excessive catecholamines, and dissection of coronary arteries. Doctors first described ACS by symptoms and pathology findings alone but over time incorporated electrocardiograms (EKGs), coronary angiography, laboratory tests of increasing sensitivity, and a host of new imaging modalities. The protocol-driven treatment of ST segment elevation myocardial infarction (STEMI) is so well-rehearsed that recognition, EKG, laboratories, and intervention in the coronary catheterization laboratory happen within 90 minutes in the United States[1] and within 60 minutes in Europe.[2]

Protocolized care improves survival and functional outcomes for men and women with many but not all the ACS pathologic conditions. A significant proportion of women

Department of Emergency Medicine, Virginia Tech Carilion School of Medicine, 3735 Franklin Road SW, Box 269, Roanoke, VA 24014, USA
* Corresponding author.
E-mail address: rmbrown@carilionclinic.org

Emerg Med Clin N Am 40 (2022) 629–636
https://doi.org/10.1016/j.emc.2022.06.003
emed.theclinics.com

with ACS suffer adverse outcomes because of an oversimplified understanding of the disease, its presentation, and its treatment. There is great urgency to correct this because the incidence of coronary artery disease (CAD) in women decreased steadily after 1968 but began rising again for the first time between 2000 and 2002.[3]

Worsening Trends in Mortality

The danger is not just an increasing incidence of ACS but increasing mortality among certain groups. Mortality from CAD has been increasing in women aged 45 to 54 years since 1999 and has been increasing in women aged 55 to 64 years since 2009. Increased mortality reflects an urban/rural divide with urban and suburban women seeing mortality improvement at the same time as a significant increase in mortality among rural white women.[4] Despite significant gains, women's mortality from cardiovascular disease has been higher than men's since 1984.[5] The proposed reasons are many.

Risk Factors Vary by Sex

There are risk factors more common in women and unique to women, which significantly increase the risk of ACS: autoimmune/inflammatory diseases, Polycystic Ovary Syndrome (PCOS), early menopause, preeclampsia, gestational diabetes, and gestational hypertension.[6] There are risk factors that disproportionately affect women, such as diabetes, which may increase the risk of ACS in women 4-fold compared with 2.5-fold in men.[7] Smoking may increase the relative risk of ACS in women more than in men (3.3 vs 1.9 in one study) and more than 7 times the relative risk in women aged 35 to 44 years.[8] Even moderate-to-severe depression correlates with a higher mortality and may be more common in women aged less than 55 years after myocardial infarction (MI).[9] The emergency physician is the critical gatekeeper charged with recognizing a host of different presentations of this family of pathologies.[10]

Unique Pathologic Condition in Women

Women have relatively smaller coronary arteries than men per unit mass[11]; a finding proposed to increase shear forces and both spare women from a greater share of obstructive CAD[12] while also causing endothelial pathologic condition, which makes women the majority of cases of nonobstructive CAD.[13] A distinct set of imaging techniques are needed to uncover it.[14] These patients are more likely to suffer non-ST elevation myocardial infarction (NSTEMI), unstable angina,[15] and MI with nonobstructive CAD.[16]

Among nonobstructive ACS cases, there are distinct patterns with men more likely to experience coronary artery spasm (Prinzmetal angina),[17] whereas women are more likely to have coronary microvascular dysfunction (CMVD).[18] Theories for the cause of CMVD include microemboli, hypertrophy-induced perivascular fibrosis, which causes compression of vessels, and overconstriction or failure of dilation of the vessels due to endothelial dysfunction.[19]

Takotsubo cardiomyopathy is yet another distinct ACS presentation with more than 88% of cases occurring in women.[20] The cause is likely sympathetic overstimulation,[21] although it primarily occurs with negative emotions.[22]

Spontaneous coronary artery dissection (SCAD) represents roughly 1% of MIs but the true rate is not known because the standard coronary angiography does not detect all cases; 90% of cases occur in women.[23] The incidence of SCAD in MI in young women may be as high as 10% to 20%.[24] Estimates of the incidence of SCAD in MI in pregnant women range from 35%[25] to 43% and typically occurs in the last trimester or the first 3 months postpartum.[26] Risk factors include multiparity and preeclampsia.[27]

Delays to Presentation and the Need for Public Recognition

It took concerted campaigns by the US government and American Heart Association to increase awareness of cardiovascular disease as the leading cause of death in women (from 30% aware in 1997% to 57% aware in 2006 but then down to 54% aware in 2009).[28] A similar effort may be needed to call attention to the many varieties of CAD which skew younger, female, and which may not present with chest pain as the most prominent symptom or a symptom at all. The time from symptom onset to intervention is even more important than the time from emergency department (ED) presentation to intervention[29] but the ED is our first chance to intervene.

Estimates suggest 8% of ACS occurs in patients less than 45 and less than 16% of these cases are women but unlike age-matched young men who have improved odds of survival compared with their older peers, women are more likely to die in this young cohort compared with older women. Compared with age-matched men, these women are 6 times more likely to die.[30] This may have to do with a delayed door to balloon time, especially in younger women.[31] Even in the case of STEMI, the most closely monitored and quality-improved of all ACS presentations, young women are less likely to receive reperfusion therapy and are more likely to be delayed when they do receive it.[32]

OBSERVATION/ASSESSMENT/EVALUATION
Presenting Symptoms Vary by Sex

Chest pain is still the most common presentation of ACS but women are more likely than men to present without chest pain (42% compared with 31% by one estimate). Age less than 45 years increases the risk of presenting without chest pain and the mortality compared with an age-matched male cohort (OR 1.18 for women aged < 45 years, although CI = 1–1.39).[33] In one retrospective study, women aged less than 55 years were more likely to present to the ED in the days to weeks before ACS with prodromal symptoms of fatigue, sleep disturbance, anxiety, and arm weakness/discomfort but even though they arrived more commonly by ambulance than their male counterparts, cardiovascular risk reduction therapy was given in less than 40% of cases.[34] Among all women with ACS presenting without chest pain, dyspnea, weakness, malaise, and pain in the neck, jaw, and upper back were reported instead.[35]

Laboratories Vary by Sex

High sensitivity troponin demonstrates sex-based differences in thresholds for ACS and early studies called for adjustments to prevent overdiagnosis in men[36] and underdiagnosis in women,[37] so that the fourth universal definition of MI now calls for different upper reference limits for men and women.[38] Male myocardium is more massive,[39] even accounting for age and body surface area.[40]

Imaging Tailored to Pathology

Women are more likely to have plaque erosions on optical coherence tomography compared with men who are more likely to have plaque rupture visible on angiography.[41] Coronary artery calcium (CAC) measured by CT shows women have fewer lesions but greater lesion size and higher plaque density, with significantly higher mortality risk associated with multivessel CAC, greater than 4 lesions, and lesions greater than 15 mm^3 when compared with men.[42] Diagnosis of CMVD requires myocardial perfusion PET scanning or invasive vasoreactivity testing and the workup may be appropriate for patients with a blunted heart rate response during pharmacologic stress testing.[43] SCAD is better diagnosed with optical coherence tomography or intravascular ultrasound.[44]

THERAPEUTIC OPTIONS
Disparities in Care

Women are less likely to be referred for coronary catheterization, percutaneous intervention, and fibrinolysis[45] and are less likely to receive secondary prevention with ACE inhibitors and antilipid medications, even after adjusting for age, comorbidities, and the physician's assessment of the risk of cardiac catheterization.[5,46] One randomized controlled trial of early, aggressive revascularization in non-ST elevation ACS demonstrated benefit for patients with NSTEMI (presenting with elevated troponin) but the composite outcome of death, MI, Cerebrovascular Accident (CVA), repeat hospitalization, or severe bleeding within 1 year is difficult to parse and requires follow-up study if this is a method to reduce mortality disparities.[47]

A study from 2010 to 2014 demonstrated women have a higher risk of in-hospital mortality after Percutaneous Intervention (PCI).[48] These short-term (30 days) mortality disparities exist after controlling for age and comorbidities but they resolve in long-term (>6 month) follow-up.[49] In part due to older age at presentation and additional comorbidities, women are more likely to die of noncardiac causes 6 years after ACS, whereas in men cardiovascular causes of death remain the most likely for any period of time following ACS.[50]

Protocols Eliminate Disparities

Implementation of the Cleveland Clinic Comprehensive 4-step STEMI protocol resolved sex disparities and improved mortality by (1) initiating cardiac catheterization laboratory activation by ED physicians without cardiology consult following activation criteria, (2) standardization of goal-directed medical therapy at triage using an STEMI checklist, (3) initiation of immediate transfer to the first open cath laboratory without delays waiting for a specific cath laboratory, and (4) radial access was chosen preferentially.[51]

Regardless of acute intervention, roughly 69% of the sex disparity in mortality could be reduced by optimizing guideline-based medical therapy at discharge after ACS.[52] Nonobstructive CAD is a unique disease, which requires unique treatment as demonstrated by a follow-up cohort, which did not benefit from dual antiplatelet therapy but did benefit from ACE inhibitors/ARBs, statins, and beta blockers.[53]

Treatment of Spontaneous Coronary Artery Dissection

Treatment of SCAD is a unique consideration. In-hospital mortality decreased over the course of one study (11.4% in 2009% to 5.0% in 2014) coinciding with a decrease in PCI (82.5%–69.1%) but note that while PCI was associated with greater mortality in cases of NSTEMI with SCAD, it was associated with improved survival in cases of STEMI with SCAD.[23] Conservative therapy with blood pressure control and beta blockers to reduce shear forces on the dissection is now recommended to permit intramural hematoma reabsorption within the month and limiting the risk of guidewire-induced dissection propagation.

SUMMARY

Women aged less than 55 years are more likely to suffer from pathologic conditions of the coronary arteries, which are distinct in presentation, laboratories, imaging, and treatment than that seen in men and older women. Higher mortality in all women is the result of a failure to recognize the many pathologic conditions within ACS and a failure to activate protocolized and guideline-directed therapy as early as possible. Using agreed-upon criteria to rapidly intervene when all patients with ACS present seems to reduce or eliminate sex disparities in mortality, as does following guideline-based recommendations for medical therapy at discharge from the hospital.

CLINICS CARE POINTS

- Acute coronary syndrome (ACS) encompasses acute thrombotic occlusion of coronary arteries as well as coronary microvascular dysfunction, coronary vasospasm, spontaneous coronary artery dissection, and Takotsubo cardiomyopathy.

- Presentations may be marked by symptoms such as fatigue, dyspnea, weakness, and pain in the jaw, neck, and upper back.

- High sensitivity troponins have different thresholds for ACS in men and women.

- Assessment with coronary angiography is appropriate with elevated troponin but assessment with coronary artery calcium score, optical coherence tomography, myocardial perfusion PET scanning, or intravascular ultrasound may be more appropriate otherwise.

- Protocolized and guideline-based care provided quickly to men and women eliminates sex disparities in mortality.

DISCLOSURE

The author has nothing to disclose.

REFERENCES

1. Levine GN, Bates ER, Bittl JA, et al. 2016 ACC/AHA Guideline Focused Update on Duration of Dual Antiplatelet Therapy in Patients With Coronary Artery Disease: A Report of the American College of Cardiology/American Heart Association Task Force on Clinical Practice Guidelines: An Update of the 2011 ACCF/AHA/SCAI Guideline for Percutaneous Coronary Intervention, 2011 ACCF/AHA Guideline for Coronary Artery Bypass Graft Surgery, 2012 ACC/AHA/ACP/AATS/PCNA/SCAI/STS Guideline for the Diagnosis and Management of Patients With Stable Ischemic Heart Disease, 2013 ACCF/AHA Guideline for the Management of ST-Elevation Myocardial Infarction, 2014 AHA/ACC Guideline for the Management of Patients With Non-ST-Elevation Acute Coronary Syndromes, and 2014 ACC/AHA Guideline on Perioperative Cardiovascular Evaluation and Management of Patients Undergoing Noncardiac Surgery. Circulation 2016;134(10):e123–55.
2. Ibanez B, James S, Agewall S, et al. 2017 ESC Guidelines for the management of acute myocardial infarction in patients presenting with ST-segment elevation: The Task Force for the management of acute myocardial infarction in patients presenting with ST-segment elevation of the European Society of Cardiology (ESC). Eur Heart J 2018;39(2):119–77.
3. Ford ES, Capewell S. Coronary heart disease mortality among young adults in the U.S. from 1980 through 2002: concealed leveling of mortality rates. J Am Coll Cardiol 2007;50(22):2128–32.
4. Bossard M, Latifi Y, Fabbri M, et al. Increasing Mortality From Premature Coronary Artery Disease in Women in the Rural United States. J Am Heart Assoc Cardiovasc Cerebrovasc Dis 2020;9(9).

5. Mehta LS, Beckie TM, DeVon HA, et al. Acute Myocardial Infarction in Women: A Scientific Statement From the American Heart Association. Circulation 2016; 133(9):916–47.

6. Young L, Cho L. Unique cardiovascular risk factors in women. Heart 2019; 105(21):1656–60.

7. Yusuf S, Hawken S, Ounpuu S, et al. Effect of potentially modifiable risk factors associated with myocardial infarction in 52 countries (the INTERHEART study): case-control study. Lancet 2004;364(9438):937–52.

8. Njolstad I, Arnesen E, Lund-Larsen PG. Smoking, serum lipids, blood pressure, and sex differences in myocardial infarction. A 12-year follow-up of the Finnmark Study. Circulation 1996;93(3):450–6.

9. Shah AJ, Ghasemzadeh N, Zaragoza-Macias E, et al. Sex and age differences in the association of depression with obstructive coronary artery disease and adverse cardiovascular events. J Am Heart Assoc 2014;3(3):e000741.

10. Haider A, Bengs S, Luu J, et al. Sex and gender in cardiovascular medicine: presentation and outcomes of acute coronary syndrome. Eur Heart J 2020;41(13): 1328–36.

11. Hiteshi AK, Li D, Gao Y, et al. Gender differences in coronary artery diameter are not related to body habitus or left ventricular mass. Clin Cardiol 2014;37(10): 605–9.

12. Kerkhof PLM, Miller VM, Wenger NK, et al. Sex-specific Analysis of cardiovascular function. Advances in Experimental medicine and Biology1065. Cham: Springer Nature; 2018. VII-VIII.

13. Lee B-K, Lim HS, Fearon WF, et al. Invasive Evaluation of Patients With Angina in the Absence of Obstructive Coronary Artery Disease. Circulation 2015;131(12): 1054–60.

14. Patel MB, Bui LP, Kirkeeide RL, et al. Imaging Microvascular Dysfunction and Mechanisms for Female-Male Differences in CAD. JACC Cardiovasc Imaging 2016;9(4):465–82.

15. Akhter N, Milford-Beland S, Roe MT, et al. Gender differences among patients with acute coronary syndromes undergoing percutaneous coronary intervention in the American College of Cardiology-National Cardiovascular Data Registry (ACC-NCDR). Am Heart J 2009;157(1):141–8.

16. Smilowitz NR, Mahajan AM, Roe MT, et al. Mortality of Myocardial Infarction by Sex, Age, and Obstructive Coronary Artery Disease Status in the ACTION Registry–GWTG (Acute Coronary Treatment and Intervention Outcomes Network Registry–Get With the Guidelines). Circ Cardiovasc Qual Outcomes 2017;10(12):1–8.

17. Kawana A, Takahashi J, Takagi Y, et al. Gender differences in the clinical characteristics and outcomes of patients with vasospastic angina–a report from the Japanese Coronary Spasm Association. Circ J : official J Jpn Circ Soc 2013;77(5): 1267–74.

18. Sara JD, Widmer RJ, Matsuzawa Y, et al. Prevalence of Coronary Microvascular Dysfunction Among Patients With Chest Pain and Nonobstructive Coronary Artery Disease. JACC: Cardiovasc Interventions 2015;8(11):1445–53.

19. Ahmed B, Creager Mark A. Alternative causes of myocardial ischemia in women: An update on spontaneous coronary artery dissection, vasospastic angina and coronary microvascular dysfunction. Vasc Med 2017;22(2):146–60.

20. Pattisapu VK, Hua H, Yunxian L, et al. Sex- and Age-Based Temporal Trends in Takotsubo Syndrome Incidence in the United States. J Am Heart Assoc 2021; 10(20):1–3.

21. Esler M. The sympathetic regulation of the heart. Eur Heart J 2016;37(37):2808–9.

22. Ghadri JR, Templin C. The InterTAK Registry for Takotsubo Syndrome. Eur Heart J 2016;37(37):2806–8.

23. Mahmoud AN, Taduru SS, Mentias A, et al. Trends of Incidence, Clinical Presentation, and In-Hospital Mortality Among Women With Acute Myocardial Infarction With or Without Spontaneous Coronary Artery Dissection: A Population-Based Analysis. JACC Cardiovasc interventions 2018;11(1):80–90.

24. Nakashima T, Noguchi T, Haruta S, et al. Prognostic impact of spontaneous coronary artery dissection in young female patients with acute myocardial infarction: A report from the Angina Pectoris-Myocardial Infarction Multicenter Investigators in Japan. Int J Cardiol 2016;207:341–8.

25. Lameijer HKM, Oudijk M. Ischaemic heart disease during pregnancy or postpartum: systematic review and case series. Neth Heart J 2015;23(5):249–57.

26. Elkayam U, Jalnapurkar S, Barakkat MN, et al. Pregnancy-Associated Acute Myocardial Infarction: A Review of Contemporary Experience in 150 Cases Between 2006 and 2011. Circulation 2014;129(16):1695–702.

27. James AH, Jamison MG, Biswas MS, et al. Acute Myocardial Infarction in Pregnancy: A United States Population-Based Study. Circulation 2006;113(12):1564–71.

28. Mosca L, Mochari-Greenberger H, Dolor RJ, et al. Sex/gender differences in cardiovascular disease prevention: what a difference a decade makes. Circulation 2011;124(19):2145–54.

29. Redfors B, Mohebi R, Giustino G, et al. Time Delay, Infarct Size, and Microvascular Obstruction After Primary Percutaneous Coronary Intervention for ST-Segment-Elevation Myocardial Infarction. Circ Cardiovasc Interv 2021;14(2):e009879.

30. Ricci B, Cenko E, Vasiljevic Z, et al. Acute Coronary Syndrome: The Risk to Young Women. J Am Heart Assoc 2017;6(12):n/a.

31. Udell JA, Fonarow GC, Maddox TM, et al. Sustained sex-based treatment differences in acute coronary syndrome care: Insights from the American Heart Association Get With The Guidelines Coronary Artery Disease Registry. Clin Cardiol 2018;41(6):758–68.

32. D'Onofrio G, Safdar B, Lichtman JH, et al. Sex differences in reperfusion in young patients with ST-segment-elevation myocardial infarction: results from the VIRGO study. Circulation 2015;131(15):1324–32.

33. Canto JG, Rogers WJ, Goldberg RJ, et al. Association of age and sex with myocardial infarction symptom presentation and in-hospital mortality. JAMA 2012;307(8):813–22.

34. Khan NA, Daskalopoulou SS, Karp I, et al. Sex differences in prodromal symptoms in acute coronary syndrome in patients aged 55 years or younger. Heart 2017;103(11):863–9.

35. Canto JG, Goldberg RJ, Hand MM, et al. Symptom Presentation of Women With Acute Coronary Syndromes: Myth vs Reality. Arch Intern Med 2007;167(22):2405–13.

36. Gore MO, Seliger SL, deFilippi CR, et al. Age- and sex-dependent upper reference limits for the high-sensitivity cardiac troponin T assay. J Am Coll Cardiol 2014;63(14):1441–8.

37. Kimenai DM, Henry RMA, van der Kallen CJ H, et al. Direct comparison of clinical decision limits for cardiac troponin T and I. Heart 2016;102(8):610–6.

38. Thygesen K, Alpert JS, Jaffe AS, et al. Fourth Universal Definition of Myocardial Infarction (2018). Circulation 2018;138(20):e618–51.

39. Salton CJ, Chuang ML, O'Donnell CJ, et al. Gender differences and normal left ventricular anatomy in an adult population free of hypertension. A cardiovascular magnetic resonance study of the Framingham Heart Study Offspring cohort. J Am Coll Cardiol 2002;39(6):1055–60.

40. Grandi AM, Venco A, Barzizza F, et al. Influence of Age and Sex on Left Ventricular Anatomy and Function in Normals. Cardiology 1992;81(1):8–13.

41. White SJ, Newby AC, Johnson TW. Endothelial erosion of plaques as a substrate for coronary thrombosis. Thromb Haemost 2016;115(03):509–19.

42. Shaw LJ, Min JK, Nasir K, et al. Sex differences in calcified plaque and long-term cardiovascular mortality: observations from the CAC Consortium. Eur Heart J 2018;39(41):3727–35.

43. Haider A, Bengs S, Maredziak M, et al. Heart rate reserve during pharmacological stress is a significant negative predictor of impaired coronary flow reserve in women. Eur J Nucl Med Mol Imaging 2019;46(6):1257–67.

44. Tamis-Holland JE, Jneid H, Reynolds HR, On behalf of the American Heart Association Interventional Cardiovascular Care Committee of the Council on Clinical, C., et al. Contemporary Diagnosis and Management of Patients With Myocardial Infarction in the Absence of Obstructive Coronary Artery Disease - A Scientific Statement From the American Heart Association. Circulation 2019;139(18): e891–908.

45. Jneid H, Fonarow GC, Cannon CP, et al. Sex Differences in Medical Care and Early Death After Acute Myocardial Infarction. Circulation 2008;118(25):2803–10.

46. Bugiardini R, Yan AT, Yan RT, on behalf of the Canadian Acute Coronary Syndrome Registry, I.a.I.I.I., et al. Factors influencing underutilization of evidence-based therapies in women. Eur Heart J 2011;32(11):1337–44.

47. Savonitto S, Cavallini C, Petronio PS, et al. *Early aggressive versus initially conservative treatment in elderly patients with non-ST-segment elevation acute coronary syndrome: a randomized controlled trial.* JACC. Cardiovasc interventions 2012;5(9):906–16.

48. Potts J, Sirker A, Martinez SC, et al. Persistent sex disparities in clinical outcomes with percutaneous coronary intervention: Insights from 6.6 million PCI procedures in the United States. PLoS ONE 2018;13(9):e0203325.

49. Bavishi C, Bangalore S, Patel D, et al. Short and long-term mortality in women and men undergoing primary angioplasty: A comprehensive meta-analysis. Int J Cardiol 2015;198:123–30.

50. Fanaroff AC, Roe MT, Clare RM, et al. Competing Risks of Cardiovascular Versus Noncardiovascular Death During Long-Term Follow-Up After Acute Coronary Syndromes. J Am Heart Assoc 2017;6(9):n/a.

51. Huded CP, Johnson M, Kravitz K, et al. 4-Step Protocol for Disparities in STEMI Care and Outcomes in Women. J Am Coll Cardiol 2018;71(19):2122–32.

52. Li S, Fonarow GC, Mukamal KJ, et al. Sex and Race/Ethnicity–Related Disparities in Care and Outcomes After Hospitalization for Coronary Artery Disease Among Older Adults. Circ Cardiovasc Qual Outcomes 2016;9(2 suppl 1):S36–44.

53. Lindahl B, Baron T, Erlinge D, et al. Medical Therapy for Secondary Prevention and Long-Term Outcome in Patients With Myocardial Infarction With Nonobstructive Coronary Artery Disease. Circulation 2017;135(16):1481–9.

The Aged Heart

Phillip D. Magidson, MD, MPH

KEYWORDS

- Geriatrics • Emergency medicine • Cardiology • Congestive heart failure
- Atrial fibrillation • Acute coronary syndrome

KEY POINTS

- Among older adults, cardiovascular disease is the leading cause of death in men and women and a leading cause for emergency department (ED) visits and acute hospitalizations.
- The management of heart failure exacerbations in older adults is similar to that in younger patients; however, for those with advanced disease, palliative care referrals should be considered in the ED.
- Older adults are more likely to present with atypical symptoms of acute coronary syndrome with more than 20% not reporting any chest pain.
- Although many older adults are at increased risk for falls, the benefits of anticoagulation in atrial fibrillation often outweigh the perceived risks. Shared decision-making should occur with patients and families before stopping blood thinners in these patients.

INTRODUCTION AND EPIDEMIOLOGY

Between 2016 and 2060, the number of adults aged 65 years and older in the United States is anticipated to increase by nearly 45 million or 92%.[1] During that same period, older adults are anticipated to go from making up 15% of the population to more than 23%.[2] This changing demographic will require the health-care system, and emergency medicine providers (EMPs), to develop specific interventions for and awareness of high value care delivery to older adults. The need for attention to cardiovascular disease (CVD) in older adults will be no exception.

The English physician Dr Thomas Sydenham is attributed with having said, "A man is as old as his arteries." Moreover, as we age, CVD increases not only in its frequency but also in severity, affecting the health-care system and the lives of older adults considerably.[3,4] Nearly 50% of adults in the United States suffer from CVD with its prevalence more likely in older adults compared with younger patients. Of older adults aged between 60 and 79 years, more than 75% had CVD with an increase to 90% in those aged 80 years and older.[5] This disease burden is associated with significant

Department of Emergency Medicine, Division of Geriatric Medicine and Gerontology, Johns Hopkins University School of Medicine, 4940 Eastern Avenue A1 East, Suite 150, Baltimore, MD 21224, USA
E-mail address: pmagidson@jhmi.edu

Emerg Med Clin N Am 40 (2022) 637–649
https://doi.org/10.1016/j.emc.2022.06.004
0733-8627/22/© 2022 Elsevier Inc. All rights reserved.
emed.theclinics.com

morbidity and mortality as CVD is the leading cause of death in men and women aged 65 years and older.[6] More than 80% of all deaths attributed to CVD are in patients aged 65 years and older.[7] Furthermore, there are considerable financial costs associated with CVD. Between 2016 and 2017, it is estimated that the United States spent nearly US$150 billion on costs related to CVD in adults aged 65 years and older.[5,8]

In the emergency department (ED), this increase burden of CVD in older adults is seen daily. The mean age for presentation to the ED with some of the most common cardiac diagnoses including acute myocardial infarction (AMI), heart failure, valvular heart disease, cardiac conduction disorder as well as atrial fibrillation (AF)/flutter is all over 65 years of age. The mean age for those patients presenting in cardiac arrest or with ventricular fibrillation/ventricular tachycardia is 63 years.[9] Although mortality among older adults with AMI has decreased during the past 2 decades, such improvement is smallest in those aged 85 years and older.[10] As EMPs, it is important to recognize this disproportionate cardiac disease burden among older adults, the reason for its existence, and how best to care for this patient population.

PATHOPHYSIOLOGY OF AGING IN CARDIOVASCULAR DISEASE

To understand heart disease among geriatric patients, we must consider 4 specific domains associated with aging: molecular, cellular, structural, and functional changes.[11]

Molecular changes found in the heart associated with aging include disruptions to mitochondrial homeostasis and increased reactive oxygen species.[12] Alterations in calcium signaling is also suggested to play a role in the development of heart failure in older adults.[11,13] Hormonal changes, especially those related to the renin-angiotensin-aldosterone system and beta adrenergic receptors, further negatively impact cardiac output and overall contractility.[14]

From a cellular standpoint, longstanding hypertension has been associated with increased fibrotic changes and collagen deposition. These changes are associated with the loss of cardiomyocytes and development of left ventricular hypertrophy.[15,16] At the atrial level, these fibrotic changes are associated with the development of atrial arrythmias such as AF.[17]

These molecular and cellular changes of aging result in structural changes that, in addition to concomitant functional changes, lead to the diseases processes that often result in ED visits among older adults.

The most striking of these structural changes include both ventricular eccentric and concentric hypertrophy as well as atrial hypertrophy with atrial dilation. These ventricular changes are key players in the development of heart failure with both reduced and preserved ejection fractions. The functional consequence of this structural change includes volume overload and similar clinical presentations often seen among older adults seen in the ED.[18,19] Furthermore, atrial structural changes described above are closely associated with AF, the most common arrythmia seen in older adults.[20]

Many of the same cellular and molecular processes also affect the development of valvular disease because the prevalence of moderate and severe mitral and aortic valvular disease increases with age. When compared with adults aged 55 to 64 years, those aged 75 years and older are nearly 5 times as likely to have mitral or aortic valvular disease.[21]

Interestingly, the development of cardiovascular structural changes, such as ventricular hypertrophy, independent of cardiovascular risk factors, comorbidities and cardiovascular medications, has been associated with cognitive decline in older adults.[22] This fact further substantiates the importance of understanding the consequences of an aging heart on the clinical and functional outcomes among older adults.

DISEASE-SPECIFIC CONSIDERATION
Hypertension and Hypertensive Emergency

Presentation: The prevalence of hypertension increases with age with approximately 70% of those aged 70 years and older having developed the disease.[23] As the most common CVD among all adults, particularly older adults, hypertension is one of the most allusive diagnoses to make, owing to the fact of its asymptomatic nature. In the ED, elevated blood pressure readings in isolation generally do not require acute intervention unless associated with end-organ dysfunction. However, many older adults are often referred to the ED for the evaluation of elevated blood pressures incidentally noted in ambulatory care sites, skilled nursing facilities, and urgent care centers. For these patients, and those with true hypertensive emergency, it is important for the EMP to know appropriate next steps when it comes to diagnostics, interventions, and referral to further care.

Diagnosis: Unlike many disease processes, the diagnosis of both hypertension and hypertensive emergencies is not uniformly clear. The American College of Cardiology/ American Heart Association (ACC/AHA) and the European Society of Cardiology/European Society of Hypertension (ESC/ESH) having different definitions of hypertension. The ACC/AHA uses blood pressure goals of less than 130/80 mm Hg, whereas their European counterparts use less than 140/90 mm Hg.[24,25] In older adults, both the ACC/AHA and ESC/ESH acknowledge that there are numerous considerations that must be made in older adults (life expectancy, frailty, cognitive impairment, adverse medication effects) when considering blood pressure goals and the decision to initiate therapy. Despite the importance of patient preference and clinical judgment when initiating blood pressure control measures in older adults, the 2015 SPRINT trial did show that even older adults (75 years of age and older) assigned to more intensive treatment goals of systolic blood pressure (<120) demonstrated lower rates of nonfatal cardiovascular events and death.[26]

The diagnosis of essential hypertension is generally not a diagnosis EMPs make because it requires numerous blood pressure readings best taken when the patient is relaxed and in a calm environment.[27] However, when elevated pressures are noted in the ED, the EMP has an obligation to encourage older adults to seek ambulatory follow-up given clear morbidity and mortality benefits associated with blood pressure control in this patient population.

Hypertensive emergency, defined as elevated blood pressures (often greater than 180/120 mm Hg) with end-organ dysfunction is not unique to older adults. End-organ dysfunction may include acute renal failure, acute coronary syndrome (ACS), aortic dissection, flash pulmonary edema, or intracranial hemorrhage. Because older adults are more prone to having elevated blood pressures, it is imperative that isolated, asymptomatic hypertension is not misclassified as hypertensive emergency simply because of an elevated systolic or diastolic reading. In the absence of clear end-organ dysfunction, rapid reduction of otherwise elevated blood pressures is associated with stroke and myocardial ischemia among older adults and should be avoided.[28,29]

Treatment: Treatment of both essential hypertension and hypertensive emergencies may be appropriate for older adults in the ED. Although the diagnosis of essential hypertension is not generally made in the ED, reinitiation of previously prescribed antihypertensive medications may be appropriate for some older adults. Still, caution should be taken when ordering these medications. Older adults may lack the ability to effectively generate a sympathetic response to physiologic stress causing them to be more sensitive to these medications, especially during times of even mild acute illness. For example, reinitiation of home antihypertensives may precipitate hypotension in septic or hypovolemic older adults that would otherwise not occur in younger patients. Additionally, orthostatic hypotension is seen in up to one-third of community-dwelling older adults and up to 50% of nursing home patients.[30,31] For this reason, patients with conditions known to exacerbate orthostatic hypotension (dehydration, prolonged bed rest, Parkinson disease) should have routine blood pressure medications held or only very slowly reintroduced in the acute setting.

Older adults being treated for hypertensive emergency should generally be given similar considerations as younger adults; however, there are some side effects and adverse reactions to consider among older adults when initiating hypertensive emergency treatment (**Table 1**).

Disposition: For older adults referred to the ED with asymptomatic hypertension, further testing is not warranted. These patients may be referred to a primary care provider for confirmatory ambulatory blood pressure measurements and/or reinitiation of home blood pressure medications.[32] For those patients undergoing the treatment of true hypertensive emergency, intensive care unit admission is often most appropriate.

Acute Coronary Syndrome

Presentation: Generally speaking, the presentation for ACS in older adults is similar to that in younger patients with a few considerations. The first is that although typical chest pain (chest squeezing, heaviness, pressure) remains the primary presenting symptom in most older adults with ACS, it is less commonly reported than in younger patients.[33,34] Atypical chest pain (burning, pleuritic or reproducible) is much more common in older adults. According to one study, up to 22% of older adults with ACS present without chest pain at all.[33] Furthermore, older adults are less likely to present within 6 hours of symptom onset as opposed to younger patients. **Table 2** summarizes differences in clinical presentation between older and younger adults diagnosed with ACS.

Diagnosis: The challenges associated with diagnosis stem more from subtleties of presentation in older adults rather than differences in diagnostic criteria. An appropriate workup for suspected ACS consists of laboratory tests including a troponin level as well as an electrocardiogram (ECG). With respect to the ECG, older adults are more likely to present with a non-ST segment elevation myocardial infarction (NSTEMI) than an ST segment elevation myocardial infarction (STEMI) when having an acute coronary event.[35,36] Additionally, older adults are more likely to have chronically elevated baseline levels of cardiac biomarker, which can further challenge EMPs attempting to determine if acute, rather than chronic, pathologic condition exists.[35,37] Elevation in brain natriuretic peptide (BNP) has been noted to be more pronounced in older adults with ACS and further predicts worse outcomes suggesting an increased diagnostic value of this marker in older patients.[38]

Treatment: The treatment of older adults with confirmed or highly suspected ACS is managed similarly to younger adults. Early, dual antiplatelet therapy with or without systemic anticoagulation should be considered. However, the risks associated with these medications, specifically bleeding, must be strongly considered in this population because they are at an increased risk of complications due to polypharmacy and numerous medical comorbidities.[35,39]

Emergent revascularization with percutaneous coronary intervention is also generally appropriate in older adults with ACS. Improved outcomes associated with early invasive strategy compared with medical therapy alone have been noted both in STEMI as well as NSTEMI older adult patients.[40,41] For this reason, the early involvement of interventional cardiologists is warranted.

Table 1
Hypertensive emergency considerations in older adults

Medication	Hypertensive Emergency Indication	Specific Geriatric Considerations
Esmolol	Often used in conjunction with other agents in aortic dissection	Caution when used in patients with bradycardia, heart failure, and COPD; very titratable with fairly short duration of action[67,68]
Fenoldopam	In patients with renal impairment	No renal adjustment is required. May be helpful in older adult patients with known chronic kidney disease
Hydralazine	Consider in patients who cannot tolerate decrease in heart rate	Poor choice in older adults due to variable effect; avoid in patients with cardiomyopathy[69,70]
Labetalol	May be used in aortic dissection or acute intracranial hemorrhage	Increased antihypertensive effect and decreased clearance in older adults. Begin infusion at lowest possible dose and cautiously titrate[71]
Nicardipine	Useful in most hypertensive emergencies in older adults	Some reports of bradycardia in older adults; metabolized by liver and should be avoided in those with liver disease[72]
Nitroglycerin	Useful in ACS and pulmonary edema	Avoid with concurrent use of phosphodiesterase inhibitors (sildenafil, tadalafil, or vardenafil), which are medications more commonly used by older adults
Sodium nitroprusside	ACS or pulmonary edema although less commonly used	Increased risk of cyanide toxicity and, when compared with other antihypertensives, higher mortality seen in older adults[73,74]

Disposition: Older adults with concerns for ACS on presentation to the ED often require hospitalization. Increased age at the time of a diagnosis of ACS is associated with an increased 1-year mortality rate and rate of rehospitalizations due cardiac and noncardiac causes.[42] In certain patients, such as hospice patients, who have concern for ACS, discharge from the ED to an appropriate community care facility might be considered once symptoms have been abated. Such decisions should be made in consultation with existing advanced directives and patient family members.

Congestive Heart Failure

Presentation: According to the Agency for Healthcare Research and Quality, heart failure is second only to sepsis as the reason for hospitalizations among those aged 75 years and older.[43] A diagnosis of congestive heart failure is associated with aging and should be considered a geriatric syndrome because the incidence doubles with each decade of life after age 65.[6] Given this, EMPs are likely to continue to see an increase in these patients in the coming decades.

Table 2
Age specific considerations in acute coronary syndrome symptomatology

ACS Symptom	Age-Specific Discussion
Typical chest pain[33,36]	Most common symptom in both younger (more than 80%) and older (just more than 50%) adults
Atypical chest pain[33]	Atypical symptoms can be seen in younger adults (just more than 10%) but is much more common in older adults (up to 30%) and especially women
Time of presentation[33]	Younger adults are more likely to present within 6 hours of symptom onset as opposed to a delayed presentation that is more common in older patients
No chest pain[33,36]	Up to 21% of older adults may present without chest pain. Less common in younger patients
Diaphoresis[33,34]	Equally common in both younger and older adults
Nausea/vomiting[33]	More common in older adults but did not reach significance in at least one study
Radiation of pain[34]	One study found radiation of pain to jaw, left arm/shoulder and back statistically more common in younger patients; Still present in up to 40% of older adults with ACS
Dyspnea[36]	Just under 50% of older adults will complain of fatigue or SOB compared with 20% in younger patient with ACS

The two primary classes of heart failure are systolic heart failure, often referred to as heart failure with reduced ejection fraction (HFrEF), and the more common diastolic heart failure, often referred to as heart failure with preserved ejection fraction (HFpEF).[44] In the clinical setting, both HFpEF and HFrEF exacerbations present similarly with reported shortness of breath, orthopnea, dyspnea on exertion, and lower extremity edema. However, older adults may also report atypical symptoms such as dizziness, fatigue, syncope, abdominal pain, and cough.[45]

Diagnosis: An acute heart failure exacerbation (AHFE) is a clinical syndrome, diagnosed based on both history as well as certain physical and diagnostic findings. Physical examination findings consistent with AHFE may include increased work of breathing, pulmonary rales or wheezing, jugular venous distention or hepatojugular reflux as well as lower extremity and abdominal edema.[46] The sensitivity and specificity associated with many of these examination findings, however, is low. For example, rales on examination have a sensitivity of 63% and specificity of 68% for AHFE.[47] As such, physical examination findings ought to be considered within the context of the history as well as other diagnostic studies.

The utility of BNP in differentiating an AHFE from other disease processes that may present similarly (eg, chronic obstructive pulmonary disease [COPD]) in older patients is questionable. BNP elevations can be seen in chronic kidney disease, pulmonary hypertension, and pulmonary embolism and may be artificially low in obese patients. Furthermore, although the sensitivity of an elevated BNP representing an AHFE has been reported to be as high as 90%, specificity is low.[48] Additionally, studies looking at the use of BNP to help differentiate causes of acute dyspnea in older adults have suggested challenges in its interpretation.[49] The EMP should consider this laboratory value within the entire clinical context and not rely on an elevation in its value to necessarily suggest AHFE in older adults.

Chest radiographs may identify acute pulmonary vascular congestion and point-of-care ultrasonography (POCUS) can be a helpful adjunct to the clinical volume assessment. Many of the findings on chest X-ray associated with AHFE such as pulmonary edema or pleural effusions can be seen in other disease processes making such findings very specific but not sensitive for AHFE.[47,50] With respect to POCUS, positive B lines is associated with a sensitivity and specificity for AHFE of 94.1% and 92.7%, respectively.[47]

Treatment: The treatment of AHFE in older adults is similar to that in younger patients. For patients presenting with pronounced hypertension and hypoxia, this may include noninvasive positive pressure ventilation strategies with or without the use of pharmacologic agents such as nitroglycerin. Diuresis may be necessary as well. Determination of a specific trigger can be helpful but it is also important to recognize congestive heart failure is a chronic disease, often with reoccurring symptoms or periods of decompensation without obvious precipitants.

Disposition: Most older adults seen in the ED for AHFE will require hospitalization. For those with recurrent presentations or advance disease, palliative care should be considered. Palliative care, or care focused on quality of life and the amelioration of symptoms, rather than a curative approach, is often thought of within the context of oncologic disease. Nevertheless, advanced CVD, particularly those patients with advanced heart failure, may benefit from early involvement of palliative care consultation.[51] The progressive nature of heart failure often means many of these patients have repeated ED visits and hospitalizations for symptom management. Despite said progressive nature and ultimate lethality associated with congestive heart failure, palliative care consultation for these patients is less common than for oncology patients.[52] Although more research in this field is needed, retrospective observational studies have suggested that earlier involvement of palliative care among heart failure patients seen in the ED should be considered.[53]

Atrial Fibrillation

Presentation: Nearly three-quarters of all patients with a diagnosis of AF are aged between 65 and 85 years. Overall, AF is the most common arrhythmia in older adults and its prevalence increases with age.[54–56] In the ED, older adults often present with complications associated with AF. These include acute strokes, serious bleeding secondary to anticoagulation or AF that is noted within the context of other acute disease processes such as infection, ACS, or heart failure exacerbation.[57] In older adults who present with dizziness, palpitations, shortness of breath, or even generalized weakness, an ECG should be obtained.

Diagnosis: The diagnosis of AF is often known before presentation to the ED; however, a new diagnosis may be made in the ED. In both instances, it is important for the EMP to understand that AF generally requires both abnormal atrial tissue giving rise to ectopic atrial beats coupled with an underlying trigger.[58,59] Many of these underlying triggers are the result of an acute treatable condition that must not be overlooked.

Treatment: Treatment of AF focuses on 3 specific domains: (1) identification and treatment of an inciting event, (2) medical management of the arrythmia itself via rate or rhythm control, and (3) prevention of thromboembolic events. For this article, we will focus on addressing the second and third domains and specific considerations among older adults.

In most instances, rate control is the preferred first-line management approach for older adults with AF. Beta blockers and nondihydropyridine calcium channel blockers are well studied in older adults and remain effective in achieving rate control. Although digoxin is recommended as a rate control agent in acute heart failure, in patients without heart failure, it has been shown to increase mortality. Additionally, dosing adjustments are necessary in renally impaired patients.[60] Although no major difference in

Table 3
Adverse Effects in older adults associated with common rhythm control agents

Rhythm Control Agent	Adverse Effect Considerations
Amiodarone	Safest rhythm control option however extracardiac side effects seen include hyper/hypothyroidism, transaminitis, optic neuropathy, and pulmonary fibrosis. QT prolongation or other conduction impairments have also been seen[75,76]
Flecainide	Associated with ventricular arrhythmias and increased mortality in patients with history of myocardial infarction[57,77]
Dofetilide	Increased arrythmias noted in patients with renal impairment. Requires dosing adjustments in said patients[57]
Dronedarone	Increased cardiovascular events seen among older adults with a history of coronary artery disease, stroke, heart failure, hypertension, and diabetes[78]
Sotalol	Increased arrythmias noted in patients with renal impairment. Requires dosing adjustments in said patients[79]

mortality has been appreciated in patients aged 65 years and older with respect to rate versus rhythm control, many rhythm control agents must be avoided in patients with comorbid liver, renal and cardiac conditions, thus making a strategy of rhythm control more complicated in older adults.[61,62] **Table 3** highlights adverse effects to consider in older adults with respect to rhythm control agents.

Prevention of thromboembolic events is a corner stone of AF management. EMPs, although perhaps not initiating anticoagulation (AC) in these patients, often must decide if such anticoagulation should be continued when an older adult presents with an acute bleeding episode or a traumatic injury. Although some literature suggests increased risk of bleeding among patients prone to falls, the risk of morbidity associated with stroke often outweighs said morbidity associated with bleeding and thus favors continued use of AC.[63] One study has suggested that a patient would need to fall nearly 300 times a year for the risk of anticoagulation to outweigh the benefit in an older adult with AF.[64] Use of risk stratification tools including HAS-BLED, HEMMORR2HAGES, and CHA2DS2-VASc coupled with shared decision-making should drive decisions on continued use of AC in older adults with AF.[65,66]

Disposition: Disposition from the ED is often related to whether a patient has established AF and/or the cause of an associated exacerbation. Older adults with known AF and a reason for an isolated complication, such as palpitations noted in a patient who has run out of their medication, may be eligible for discharge after resumption of home medications. Conversely, new onset AF in an older adult or those with serious, acute underlying pathologic condition triggering AF often requires hospitalization.

SUMMARY

CVD among older adults is common. Although the specific conditions seen in older adults may be similar to that in younger patients, the structural and functional changes of aging result in presentation subtleties, diagnostic nuances, and treatment differences among geriatric patients who present to the ED with CVD. EMPs will benefit from recognizing these differences as the population ages and the frequency in which geriatric CVD is encountered in the ED setting continues to increase.

CLINICS CARE POINTS

- Isolated, asymptomatic hypertension does not require acute treatment in the ED and should be referred to ambulatory providers for further management.
- Fatigue, shortness of breath, nausea and vomiting as well as atypical chest pain is much more common in older adults presenting with ACS than younger patients.
- Over 20% of older adults with ACS will present without chest pain.
- Palliative care should be engaged early for older adults with repeat ED visits for decompensated CHF.
- The risks associated with anticoagulation (AC) are often outweighed by the benefits seen in older adults with atrial fibrillation. Generally, AC should not be discontinued because of non-injurious fall.

DISCLOSURE

None.

REFERENCES

1. United States census bureau. an aging nation: projected number of children and older adults. 2018. Available at: https://www.census.gov/library/visualizations/2018/comm/historic-first.html. Accessed August 9, 2021.
2. Vespa J, Medina L, Armstrong D. Demographic turning points for the United States: population projections for 2020 to 2060. 2020. Available at: https://census.gov/programs-surveys/popproj.html. Accessed August 9, 2021.
3. Dodson JA, Matlock DD, Forman DE. Geriatric cardiology: an emerging discipline. Can J Cardiol 2016;32(9):1056–64. https://doi.org/10.1016/j.cjca.2016.03.019.
4. National Institute of Health. Aging hearts and arteries: a scientific quest. 2005. Available at: https://g5-assets-cld-res.cloudinary.com/image/upload/v1556125047/g5/g5-c-iqbdy3ug-terrace-communities-client/uploads/Aging_Hearts_and_Arteries_y0lf0j.pdf. Accessed August 21, 2021.
5. Virani SS, Alonso A, Aparicio HJ, et al. Heart disease and stroke statistics-2021 update a report from the american heart association. Circulation 2021;143(8): E254–743.
6. Mozaffarian D, Benjamin EJ, Go AS, et al. Heart disease and stroke statistics-2016 update a report from the american heart association 2016;133. https://doi.org/10.1161/CIR.0000000000000350.
7. Lloyd-Jones D, Adams R, Carnethon M, et al. Heart disease and stroke statistics—2009 update. Circulation 2009;119(3). https://doi.org/10.1161/circulationaha.108.191261.
8. Agency for Healthcare Research and Quality. Household component summary table. 2021. Available at: https://meps.ahrq.gov/mepstrends/home/index.html. Accessed August 21, 2021.
9. Kwok CS, Wong CW, Ravindran R, et al. Location of death among patients presenting with cardiovascular disease to the emergency department in the United states. Int J Clin Pract 2021;75(4):1–9.
10. Krumholz HM, Normand SLT, Wang Y. Twenty-year trends in outcomes for older adults with acute myocardial infarction in the United States. JAMA Netw open 2019;2(3):e191938.

11. Steenman M, Lande G. Cardiac aging and heart disease in humans. Biophys Rev 2017;9(2):131–7.
12. Tocchi A, Quarles EK, Basisty N, et al. Mitochondrial dysfunction in cardiac aging. Biochim Biophys Acta - Bioenerg 2015;1847(11):1424–33.
13. Meyer M, Schillinger W, Pieske B, et al. Alterations of sarcoplasmic reticulum proteins in failing human dilated cardiomyopathy. Circulation 1995;92(4):778–84.
14. Orsborne C, Chaggar PS, Shaw SM, et al. The renin-angiotensin-aldosterone system in heart failure for the non-specialist: the past, the present and the future. Postgrad Med J 2017;93(1095):29–37.
15. Keller KM, Howlett SE. Sex differences in the biology and pathology of the aging heart. Can J Cardiol 2016;32(9):1065–73.
16. Song Y, Yao Q, Zhu J, et al. Age-related variation in the interstitial tissues of the cardiac conduction system; and autopsy study of 230 Han Chinese. Forensic Sci Int 1999;104(2–3):133–42. https://doi.org/10.1016/S0379-0738(99)00103-6.
17. Burstein B, Nattel S. Atrial Fibrosis: Mechanisms and Clinical Relevance in Atrial Fibrillation. J Am Coll Cardiol 2008;51(8):802–9. https://doi.org/10.1016/j.jacc.2007.09.064.
18. Velagaleti RS, Gona P, Pencina MJ, et al. Left ventricular hypertrophy patterns and incidence of heart failure with preserved versus reduced ejection fraction. Am J Cardiol 2014;113(1):117–22.
19. Katz AM, Rolett EL. Heart failure: When form fails to follow function. Eur Heart J 2016;37(5):449–54.
20. Lam CSP, Rienstra M, Tay WT, et al. Atrial fibrillation in heart failure with preserved ejection fraction: association with exercise capacity, left ventricular filling pressures, natriuretic peptides, and left atrial volume. JACC Hear Fail 2017;5(2):92–8.
21. Nkomo VT, Gardin JM, Skelton TN, et al. Burden of valvular heart diseases: a population-based study. Lancet 2006;368(9540):1005–11.
22. Mahinrad S, Vriend AE, Jukema JW, et al. Left ventricular hypertrophy and cognitive decline in old age. J Alzheimer's Dis 2017;58(1):275–83.
23. Franklin SS, Larson MG, Khan SA, et al. Does the relation of blood pressure to coronary heart disease risk change with aging?: the Framingham Heart Study. Circulation 2001;103(9):1245–9.
24. Williams B, Mancia G, Spiering W, et al. 2018 ESC/ESH Guidelines for the management of arterial hypertension: The task force for the management of arterial hypertension of the european society of cardiology (ESC) and the European Society of Hypertension (ESH). Eur Heart J 2018;39(33):3021–104. https://doi.org/10.1093/eurheartj/ehy339.
25. Whelton PK, Carey RM, Aronow WS, et al. 2017 *ACC/AHA/AAPA/ABC/ACPM/AGS/APhA/ASH/ASPC/NMA/PCNA Guideline for the Prevention*, detection, evaluation, and management of high blood pressure in adults: executive summary: a Report of the American College of Cardiology/American Heart Association Task 2018;71. https://doi.org/10.1161/HYP.0000000000000066.
26. SPRINT Research Group, Wright JT Jr, Williamson JD, et al. A randomized trial of intensive versus standard blood-pressure control. N Engl J Med 2015;373(22):2103–16.
27. Shimbo D, Artinian NT, Basile JN, et al. Self-measured blood pressure monitoring at home: a joint policy statement from the american heart association and american medical association. Circulation 2020;142(4):E42–63.
28. Fischberg GM, Lozano E, Rajamani K, et al. Stroke precipitated by moderate blood pressure reduction. J Emerg Med 2000;19(4):339–46.

29. Weder AB, Erickson S. Treatment of hypertension in the inpatient setting: use of intravenous labetalol and hydralazine. J Clin Hypertens 2010;12(1):29–33.
30. Chester JG, Rudolph JL. Vital signs in older patients: age-related changes. J Am Med Dir Assoc 2011;12(5):337–43.
31. Lipsitz LA. Orthostatic hypotension in the elderly. N Engl J Med 1989;321(14): 952–7.
32. Wolf SJ, Lo B, Shih RD, et al. Clinical policy: critical issues in the evaluation and management of adult patients in the emergency department with asymptomatic elevated blood pressure. Ann Emerg Med 2013;62(1):59–68.
33. Bhatia LC, Naik RH. Clinical profile of acute myocardial infarction in elderly patients. J Cardiovasc Dis Res 2013;4(2):107–11.
34. Solomon CG, Lee TH, Cook EF, et al. Comparison of clinical presentation of acute myocardial infarction in patients older than 65 years of age to younger patients: The multicenter chest pain study experience. Am J Cardiol 1989;63(12):772–6. https://doi.org/10.1016/0002-9149(89)90040-4.
35. Dai X, Busby-Whitehead J, Alexander KP. Acute coronary syndrome in the older adults. J Geriatr Cardiol 2016;13(2):101–8.
36. Goch A, Misiewicz P, Rysz J, et al. The clinical manifestation of myocardial infarction in elderly patients. Clin Cardiol 2009;32(6):E46–51.
37. Alpert JS, Thygesen KA, White HD, et al. Diagnostic and therapeutic implications of type 2 myocardial infarction: review and commentary. Am J Med 2014;127(2): 105–8.
38. Morrow DA, De Lemos JA, Sabatine MS, et al. Evaluation of B-type natriuretic peptide for risk assessment in unstable angina/non-ST-elevation myocardial infarction: B-type natriuretic peptide and prognosis in TACTICS-TIMI 18. J Am Coll Cardiol 2003;41(8):1264–72.
39. Andreotti F, Rocca B, Husted S, et al. Antithrombotic therapy in the elderly: expert position paper of the European society of cardiology working group on thrombosis. Eur Heart J 2015;36(46):3238–49.
40. Bach RG, Cannon CP, Weintraub WS. The effect of routine, early invasive management on outcome for elderly patients with non-ST-segment elevation acute coronary syndromes. ACC Curr J Rev 2004;13(11):53–4.
41. Dzavik V, Sleeper LA, Cocke TP, et al. Early revascularization is associated with improved survival in elderly patients with acute myocardial infarction complicated by cardiogenic shock: a report from the SHOCK Trial Registry. Eur Heart J 2003; 24(9):828–37.
42. Lopes RD, Gharacholou SM, Holmes DN, et al. Cumulative incidence of death and rehospitalization among the elderly in the first year after NSTEMI. Am J Med 2015;128(6):582–90.
43. Agency for Healthcare Research and Quality. HCUP Fast Stats. Healthcare cost and utilization project (HCUP). 2021. Available at: https://www.hcup-us.ahrq.gov/faststats/NationalDiagnosesServlet?year1=2018&characteristic1=25&included1=1&year2=&characteristic2=0&included2=1&expansionInfoState=hide&dataTablesState=hide&definitionsState=hide&exportState=hide. Accessed December 21, 2021.
44. Butrous H, Hummel SL. Heart failure in older adults. Can J Cardiol 2016;32(9): 1140–7.
45. Panjrath G, Ahmed A. Diagnosis and management of heart failure in older adults. Heart Fail Clin 2017;13(3):427–44.
46. Theophanous R, Huang W, Ragsdale L. Cardiopulmonary emergencies in older adults. Emerg Med Clin North Am 2021;39(2):323–38.

47. Long B, Koyfman A, Gottlieb M. Diagnosis of acute heart failure in the emergency department: an evidence-based review. West J Emerg Med 2019;20(6):875–84.

48. McCullough PA, Nowak RM, McCord J, et al. B-type natriuretic peptide and clinical judgment in emergency diagnosis of heart failure: analysis from Breathing Not Properly (BNP) Multinational Study. Circulation 2002;106(4):416–22.

49. Fabbian F, De Giorgi A, Pala M, et al. Elevated NT-proBNP levels should be interpreted in elderly patients presenting with dyspnea. Eur J Intern Med 2011;22(1): 108–11.

50. Martindale JL, Wakai A, Collins SP, et al. Diagnosing acute heart failure in the emergency department: a systematic review and meta-analysis. Acad Emerg Med 2016;23(3):223–42.

51. von Schwarz ER, He M, Bharadwaj P. Palliative care issues for patients with heart failure. JAMA Netw Open 2020;3(2):e200011.

52. Liu AY, O'Riordan DL, Marks AK, et al. A comparison of hospitalized patients with heart failure and cancer referred to palliative care. JAMA Netw Open 2020;3(2): e200020.

53. Lipinski M, Eagles D, Fischer LM, et al. Heart failure and palliative care in the emergency department. Emerg Med J 2018;35(12):726–9.

54. Kistler PM, Sanders P, Fynn SP, et al. Electrophysiologic and electroanatomic changes in the human atrium associated with age. J Am Coll Cardiol 2004; 44(1):109–16.

55. Go AS, Hylek EM, Phillips KA, et al. Prevalence of diagnosed atrial fibrillation in adults. JAMA 2001;285(18):2370.

56. Lakshminarayan K, Solid CA, Collins AJ, et al. Atrial fibrillation and stroke in the general medicare population: a 10-year perspective (1992 to 2002). Stroke 2006;37(8):1969–74.

57. Karamichalakis N, Letsas KP, Vlachos K, et al. Managing atrial fibrillation in the very elderly patient: challenges and solutions. Vasc Health Risk Manag 2015; 11:555–62.

58. Zathar Z, Karunatilleke A, Fawzy AM, et al. Atrial fibrillation in older people: concepts and controversies. Front Med 2019. https://doi.org/10.3389/fmed.2019. 00175.

59. Staerk L, Sherer JA, Ko D, et al. Atrial fibrillation: epidemiology, pathophysiology, clinical outcomes. Circ Res 2017;120(9):1501–17.

60. Hallberg P, Lindbäck J, Lindahl B, et al. Digoxin and mortality in atrial fibrillation: a prospective cohort study. Eur J Clin Pharmacol 2007;63(10):959–71.

61. Olshansky B, Rosenfeld LE, Warner AL, et al. The Atrial Fibrillation Follow-up Investigation of Rhythm Management (AFFIRM) study: approaches to control rate in atrial fibrillation. J Am Coll Cardiol 2004;43(7):1201–8.

62. Roy D, Talajic M, Nattel S, et al. Rhythm control versus rate control for atrial fibrillation and heart failure. N Engl J Med 2008;358(25):2667–77.

63. Gage BF, Birman-Deych E, Kerzner R, et al. Incidence of intracranial hemorrhage in patients with atrial fibrillation who are prone to fall. Am J Med 2005;118(6): 612–7.

64. Man-Son-Hing M, Nichol G, Lau A, et al. Choosing antithrombotic therapy for elderly patients with atrial fibrillation who are at risk for falls. Arch Intern Med 1999;159(7):677–85.

65. Pisters R, Lane DA, Nieuwlaat R, et al. A novel user-friendly score (HAS-BLED) to assess 1-year risk of major bleeding in patients with atrial fibrillation: the Euro Heart Survey. Chest 2010;138(5):1093–100.

66. Gage BF, Yan Y, Milligan PE, et al. Clinical classification schemes for predicting hemorrhage: results from the National Registry of Atrial Fibrillation (NRAF). Am Heart J 2006;151(3):713–9.
67. Sarafidis PA, Georgianos PI, Malindretos P, et al. Pharmacological management of hypertensive emergencies and urgencies: Focus on newer agents. Expert Opin Investig Drugs 2012;21(8):1089–106.
68. Alshami A, Romero C, Avila A, et al. Management of hypertensive crises in the elderly. J Geriatr Cardiol 2018;15(7):504–12.
69. Powers DR, Papadakos PJ, Wallin JD. Parenteral hydralazine revisited. J Emerg Med 1998;16(2):191–6.
70. Ludden TM, Shepherd AMM, McNay JL, et al. Hydralazine kinetics in hypertensive patients after intravenous administration. Clin Pharmacol Ther 1980;28(6): 736–42.
71. Abernethy DR, Schwartz JB, Plachetka JR, et al. Comparison in young and elderly patients of pharmacodynamics and disposition of labetalol in systemic hypertension. Am J Cardiol 1987;60(8):697–702.
72. Abboud ME, Frasure SE. Bradycardia caused by intravenous nicardipine in an elderly patient with acute ischemic infarct. Am J Emerg Med 2016;34(4): 761.e1–2.
73. Aronson S, Dyke CM, Stierer KA, et al. The ECLIPSE trials: Comparative studies of clevidipine to nitroglycerin, sodium nitroprusside, and nicardipine for acute hypertension treatment in cardiac surgery patients. Anesth Analg 2008;107(4): 1110–21.
74. Rindone JP, Sloane EP. Cyanide toxicity from sodium nitroprusside: risks and management. Ann Pharmacother 1992;26(4):515–9.
75. Trohman RG, Sharma PS, McAninch EA, et al. Amiodarone and thyroid physiology, pathophysiology, diagnosis and management. Trends Cardiovasc Med 2019;29(5):285–95.
76. Papiris SA, Triantafillidou C, Kolilekas L, et al. Amiodarone: review of pulmonary effects and toxicity. Drug Saf 2010;33(7):539–58.
77. Echt DS, Liebson PR, Mitchell LB, et al. Mortality and morbidity in patients receiving encainide, flecainide, or placebo. The Cardiac Arrhythmia Suppression Trial. N Engl J Med 1991;324(12):781–8.
78. Connolly SJ, Camm AJ, Halperin JL, et al. Dronedarone in high-risk permanent atrial fibrillation. N Engl J Med 2011;365(24):2268–76.
79. Rabatin A, Snider MJ, Boyd JM, et al. Safety of twice daily sotalol in patients with renal impairment: a single center, retrospective review. J Atr Fibrillation 2018; 11(3):2047.

Hereditary Syndromes of Sudden Cardiac Death

Jeremy G. Berberian, MD

KEYWORDS

- Arrhythmogenic right ventricular cardiomyopathy
- Arrhythmogenic right ventricular dysplasia • Brugada syndrome
- Cardiogenic syncope • Epsilon waves • Hypertrophic cardiomyopathy
- Hypertrophic obstructive cardiomyopathy • Long QT syndrome

KEY POINTS

- The hereditary syndromes associated with sudden cardiac death include arrhythmogenic right ventricular cardiomyopathy, Brugada syndrome, hypertrophic obstructive cardiomyopathy, and long QT syndrome. The characteristic ECG findings for these syndromes includes:
- ARVC- epsilon waves, but T-wave inversions and prolonged S-wave upstroke $\geq$ 55 msec in leads V1-V3 are more common
- Brugada syndrome- complete or incomplete RBBB pattern with coved STE $\geq$ 2 mm followed by a negative T-wave in $\geq$ 1 of leads V1-V2
- Hypertrophic obstructive cardiomyopathy-high voltages with ST-segment and T-wave changes consistent with LVH
- Long QT syndrome- QTc interval $\geq$ 460 msec for women and $\geq$ 450 msec for men; increased risk for torsades de pointes with QTc > 500 msec

INTRODUCTION

Sudden cardiac death (SCD) describes the unexpected natural death from a cardiac cause within a short time period, generally 1 hour or lesser from the onset of symptoms, often due to a cardiac dysrhythmia.[1] Overall, the most common cause of SCD is coronary artery disease but for patients aged younger than 35 years, the most common cause of SCD is a dysrhythmia in the absence of ischemic heart disease. This article will review the background, diagnosis, and management of the common hereditary channelopathies and cardiomyopathies associated with an increased risk of SCD. These conditions include arrhythmogenic right ventricular cardiomyopathy (ARVC), Brugada syndrome (BrS), hypertrophic cardiomyopathy (HCM), and long QT syndrome (LQTS).

Department of Emergency Medicine, Christiana Care, 4755 Ogletown Stanton Road, Newark, DE 19718, USA
E-mail address: Jgberberian@gmail.com

Emerg Med Clin N Am 40 (2022) 651–662
https://doi.org/10.1016/j.emc.2022.06.005
0733-8627/22/© 2022 Elsevier Inc. All rights reserved.

Arrhythmogenic Right Ventricular Cardiomyopathy

Clinics care points

- Arrhythmogenic right ventricular cardiomyopathy is an inherited cardiomyopathy associated with sudden cardiac death due to ventricular dysrhythmias
- Diagnosis is based on the presence of structural abnormalities, histologic findings, ECG findings, and family history
- ECG findings include the following:
  - T-wave inversions in leads V1-V3 in the absence of right bundle branch block
  - Epsilon waves and/or QRS complex duration greater than 110 milliseconds in leads V1-V3
  - Left bundle branch block type ventricular tachycardia
- Long-term management includes oral beta-blockers, placement of an implantable cardiac defibrillator

INTRODUCTION

ARVC, also called arrhythmogenic right ventricular dysplasia, is an inherited cardiomyopathy associated with sudden cardiac death due to ventricular dysrhythmias. It is a progressive disease primarily of the right ventricle where myocardium is replaced by fibrous and adipose tissue leading to structural and functional abnormalities. Left ventricular involvement is typically seen later in the disease progression but can be present initially. The prevalence of ARVC in the general population is approximately 1 in 1,000 to 5,000 with an increased prevalence in Greece and Italy.[1] It is more common in men than in women. It accounts for 5% to 10% of unexplained SCDs in individuals aged younger than 65 years and is the leading cause of SCD in young people after HCM.[2]

Presentation

Patients with ARVC usually manifest symptoms between the second to fifth decades of life. ARVC is a progressive disease with varying clinical presentations depending on the stage of the disease. Common symptoms seen early in the disease process include palpitations, syncope, and dizziness or lightheadedness. Later in the disease process, the clinical presentation is consistent with biventricular heart failure that mimics a dilated cardiomyopathy. The risk of SCD is independent of the disease progression and can occur at any time and be the initial manifestation of the disease.

Diagnosis

The diagnostic criteria for ARVC includes the presence of structural abnormalities, histologic findings, ECG findings (**Fig. 1**), and family history. For the EM physician, the ECG criteria that are of particular importance include the following:[3,4]

1. T-wave inversions in leads V1-V3 in the absence of right bundle branch block in patients aged older than 14-years (seen in 85% of patients).
2. Epsilon waves in leads V1-V3 (most specific finding but only seen in 30% of patients).
3. QRS complex duration greater than 110 milliseconds in leads V1-V3.
4. Prolonged S-wave upstroke 55 milliseconds or greater in leads V1-V3 (seen in 95% of patients).
5. Left bundle branch block type ventricular tachycardia.

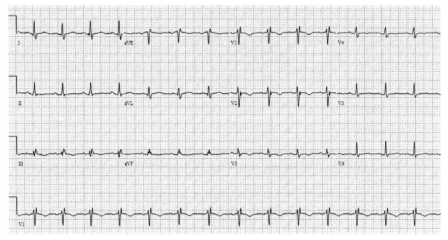

Fig. 1. ECG from a patient with ARVC. (*Courtesy of* Amal Mattu, MD.)

The epsilon wave is a low amplitude positive deflection at the end of the QRS complex that represents delayed right ventricular activation. Use of the Fontaine lead placement (**Fig. 2**) can increase the sensitivity of detection of epsilon waves up to 66%.[5] This entails placing the left arm lead on xyphoid process, the right arm lead on the manubrium, and the left leg lead in the fifth intercostal space at the midclavicular line (ie, where lead V4 is placed in a standard 12-lead ECG). The ECG should be recorded at double speed and voltage. Potential epsilon waves can be seen in leads I, II, and III (which are renamed become FI, FII, and FIII, respectively).

Management

Acute management involves the treatment of ventricular tachycardias. Patients with ARVC are often adrenergic dependent and are managed with activity restriction and

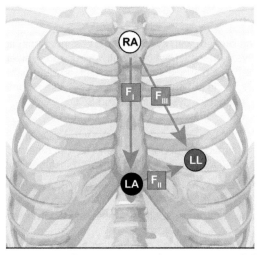

Fig. 2. Fontaine lead placement. (Image courtesy of EMRA EKG Guide.)

beta-blockers, in particular sotalol or amiodarone,[2] to reduce the frequency of dysrhythmias. Patients at high risk for SCD (eg, cardiac arrest, dysrhythmias not controlled pharmacologically) warrant placement of an implantable cardiac defibrillator. For patients who are asymptomatic and identified incidentally, disposition should be made in consultation with a cardiologist as the first manifestation of ARVC can be SCD.

Brugada Syndrome

Clinics care points

- Brugada syndrome is a sodium channelopathy that can lead to unprovoked dysrhythmias (polymorphic ventricular tachycardia or ventricular fibrillation) and cardiac arrest
- Diagnosis made from both ECG and clinical criteria
  - Type 1 is the only ECG abnormality that is potentially diagnostic
  - Type 2 is nondiagnostic but may warrant further investigation in the appropriate clinical situation
  - Type 3 is no longer considered useful in diagnosis
- Up to 40% of patients with Brugada syndrome will have normal resting ECGs
- Long-term management is placement of an implantable cardiac defibrillator

INTRODUCTION

The BrS is an autosomal dominant inherited disorder associated with an increased risk of SCD due to ventricular fibrillation (VF). The classic teaching is that BrS is a sodium channelopathy associated with a structurally normal heart but current research has identified involvement of calcium and potassium channel genes as well as minor structural abnormalities in patients with BrS.[6] BrS is thought to be responsible for 4% to 12% of all SCDs.[7] The prevalence is estimated to be between 1 in 2,000 and 1 in 5,000, and it is 8 to 10 times more prevalent in men than in women for those aged 16 years and older.[2] The mean age of BrS patients presenting with episodes of VF episodes is 41 ± 15 years but has been described in patients aged as young as 2 days.[7] The diagnosis of BrS is based on both ECG and clinical criteria.

Presentation

Patients with BrS can present with syncope, seizures, nocturnal agonal respirations, or SCD due to VF. Dysrhythmias most frequently occur during sleep or rest, often between 12 AM and 6 AM,[8] which suggest that high vagal tone and/or bradycardia may be a trigger for dysrhythmias in patients with BrS. Fever is also a common trigger of BrS and can precipitate ventricular dysrhythmias and SCD.

Diagnosis

The diagnosis of BrS is made from both ECG and clinical criteria (**Table 1**).
    The original Brugada ECG criteria set forth in 2002[9] included 3 types:

- Type 1: Coved STE 2 mm or greater followed by a negative T-wave in greater than 1 of leads V1-V3 (**Fig. 3**)
- Type 2: 2 mm or greater of saddleback shaped STE in greater than 1 of leads V1-V3
- Type 3: Type 1 or 2 morphology not meeting above criteria in greater than 1 of leads V1-V3

Table 1	
Diagnostic criteria for Brugada syndrome	
ECG Criteria	**Clinical Criteria (Must Have ≥1):**
• Complete or incomplete RBBB pattern with coved STE ≥ 2 mm followed by a negative T-wave in ≥ 1 of leads V1-V2	• Documented VF or polymorphic VT • Family history of SCD at age younger than 45 years • Coved-type ECG in family members • Inducibility of VT with programmed electrical stimulation • Syncope • Nocturnal agonal respiration

More recent 2013 guidelines[10] narrowed the definition to "Brugada syndrome is diagnosed in patients with ST-segment elevation with type 1 morphology ≥2 mm in ≥1 lead in the right precordial leads V1-V2, positioned in the 2nd, 3rd, or 4th intercostal space occurring either spontaneously or after provocative drug test with intravenous administration of class I antiarrhythmic drugs."

The important changes in the new definition include the following:
1. Type 1 is the only potentially diagnostic pattern
2. Type 1 only needs to be seen in one lead and can be seen in lead(s) V1/V2 when positioned higher than the traditional fourth intercostal space
3. Type 2 is nondiagnostic, and it is only clinically significant if the type I pattern is seen or can be provoked with sodium channel blocking antidysrhythmic medications

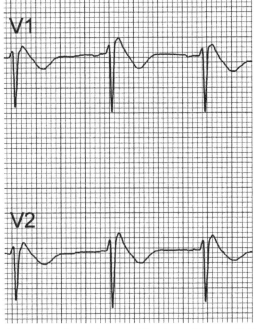

Fig. 3. Brugada syndrome type 1 morphology. (*Courtesy of* Jeremy G. Berberian, MD.)

4. Type 3 is no longer part of the criteria
5. Lead V3 is no longer part of the criteria

There are multiple conditions which can mimic the BrS type 1 pattern on the ECG (**Box 1**), so it is essential that other causes of the ECG changes are excluded before diagnosing BrS. Positioning leads V1 and V2 in the second or third intercostal space increases the sensitivity for detecting BrS type 1 pattern and can help differentiate it from a mimic. Conversely, inadvertent placement of leads V1 and V2 in the second or third intercostal spaces can produce a BrS type 2 pattern mimic in young athletes.

Management

Long-term treatment of symptomatic patients is placement of an implantable cardiac defibrillator.[5] There is no effective drug therapy to treat BrS; however, for the treatment of patients with known BrS and recurrent VF and ICD shocks, consider isoproterenol to suppress VF.[11] Quinidine may also be beneficial in treating electrical storm but is not available in many countries. Sodium channel blockers such as procainamide and flecainide should be avoided in the treatment of any patient with known or suspected BrS. Fever should be treated if present. For patients who are asymptomatic but have ECG findings, disposition should be made in consultation with a cardiologist as the first manifestation of BrS can be SCD.

Hypertrophic Cardiomyopathy

Clinics care points

- Hypertrophic cardiomyopathy (HCM) is genetic disorder characterized by ventricular hypertrophy leading to diastolic dysfunction, preload dependence, and dysrhythmias
- HCM can be suggested by clinical presentation and ECG but diagnosis is made by Doppler echocardiography or cardiac MRI
- ECG will often show changes consistent with LVH
  - Deep narrow Q-waves in the inferior and lateral leads are specific but not sensitive for HCM

Box 1
Conditions that can mimic the Brugada syndrome type 1 ECG pattern

- ARVC
- Hyperkalemia
- Immediately postelectrical cardioversion
- LAD occlusion
- Left ventricular hypertrophy
- Medications and drugs (eg, antihistamines, cocaine, fluoxetine, lithium, propofol, tricyclic antidepressants, trifluoperazine)
- Pectus excavatum
- Pulmonary embolism (acute)
- RV ischemia/infarction
- Septal hypertrophy

- Management for patients with HCM presenting in extremis should be focused on maximizing preload and afterload and treating dysrhythmias

INTRODUCTION

HCM is genetic disorder characterized by ventricular hypertrophy in the absence of an identifiable cause such as hypertension or aortic valve stenosis.[12] The incidence of HCM in the general population is estimated to be 0.2% with most patients being asymptomatic. The most common age of presentation is the third decade of life, and it is the most common cause of SCD in the young.[12] The pathophysiology of HCM is multifactorial and includes aortic outflow obstruction due to septal hypertrophy, mitral regurgitation, diastolic dysfunction, demand ischemia, dysrhythmias, and autonomic dysfunction.

Presentation

Common symptoms include dyspnea, syncope, palpitations, chest pain, dizziness, and fatigue, which can occur with exertion or at rest. The initial presentation for some patients with HCM can be SCD. Most patients with HCM are completely asymptomatic and are diagnosed because of screening. Many patients with HCM will have a systolic murmur that increases with any provocative maneuver that decreases preload (eg, Valsalva) and decreases with any provocative maneuver that increases preload (eg, Trendelenburg position). HCM predisposes patients to a variety of dysrhythmias, including atrial fibrillation, ventricular tachycardia (sustained and nonsustained), and VF. It is important to note that SCD due to a malignant dysrhythmia can occur at any time, even in patients without a history of any significant dysrhythmias.

Diagnosis

HCM can be suggested by history and ECG but it is ultimately diagnosed with Doppler echocardiography or cardiac MRI. ECG abnormalities are seen in up to 90% of patients with HCM and include the following:[13]

- High voltages with ST-segment and T-wave changes consistent with the LVH strain pattern (most common)
- Deep narrow Q-waves in the inferior and lateral leads
- Tall R-waves in the right precordial leads

HCM will often mimic the findings seen with the LVH strain pattern, in particular the large R-waves and inverted T-waves with characteristic asymmetric morphology in the lateral leads (**Fig. 4**). Although the presence of deep narrow Q-waves in the inferior and lateral leads is characteristic of HCM, their absence does not rule out HCM.

Management

Long-term management for patients with HCM is symptom-based and includes both pharmacologic and surgical treatments. Acutely, patients with HCM can present in extremis with hypotension, pulmonary edema, and tachycardia commonly due to uncontrolled atrial fibrillation. Management should be focused on maximizing preload and afterload and treating dysrhythmias. For patients presenting in uncontrolled atrial fibrillation, this can be done using intravenous beta-blockers in combination with a vasoconstrictor such as phenylephrine.[12] For patients presenting with ventricular dysrhythmias, intravenous amiodarone can be used. Aggressive diuresis or use of nitrates should be avoided because it decreases preload with can worsen the outflow obstruction. Traditional stroke scoring systems (ie, CHA_2DS_2-VASc) are not applicable to

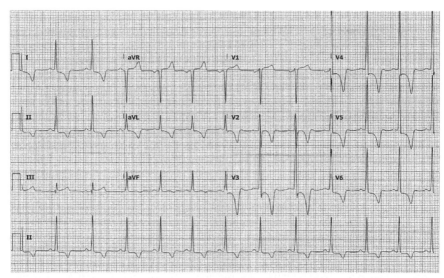

Fig. 4. The ECG of a 30-year-old man with HCM. (*Courtesy of* Jeremy G. Berberian, MD.)

patients with HCM, so anticoagulation is recommended for any patient with HCM presenting with new onset atrial fibrillation.[12] For patients who are asymptomatic and identified incidentally or because of screening, disposition should be made in consultation with a cardiologist because the first manifestation of HCM can be SCD.

Long QT Syndrome

Clinics care points

- Long QT syndrome is characterized by a prolongation of the QT interval on the ECG and increased risk of torsades de pointes (TdP)
  - Can be congenital or acquired
- Prolonged QTc interval is defined 460 milliseconds or greater for women and 450 milliseconds or greater for men
  - Increased risk for TdP typically occurs with QTc greater than 500 milliseconds
  - Manually validate the computer-generated QTc intervals on serial ECGs
- Treatment of TdP includes unsynchronized cardioversion as needed, administration of intravenous magnesium, correction of hypokalemia if present, and removal of any QT prolonging drugs
  - Electrical overdrive pacing can be used for cases refractory to pharmacologic treatment
- Long-term management includes oral beta-blockers, left cardiac sympathetic denervation, and placement of an implantable cardiac defibrillator

INTRODUCTION

Congenital LQTS is an inherited disorder that represents a leading cause of SCD in the young. It is characterized by a prolongation of the QT interval on the ECG (ie, it is a disorder of ventricular repolarization) and increased risk of torsades de pointes (TdP). Patients with congenital LQTS often have a cardiac event before 12 years of age, and the initial event can be SCD. When untreated, symptomatic patients have a mortality rate of 21% from initial syncopal episode but this is decreased to an approximately 1% 15-year mortality when properly treated.[14] LQTS can be also acquired due noninherited causes (**Box 2**).

Presentation

Patients with LQTS commonly present with syncope, seizure-like episodes, and SCD. These events are often triggered by emotional or physical stress. The dysrhythmia associated with the cardiac events of LQTS is TdP, a type of polymorphic ventricular tachycardia associated with a prolonged QTc interval on baseline ECG. It is triggered when a PVC occurs at the same time as the T-wave associated with the previous QRS complex, called "R-on-T phenomenon" (**Fig. 5**).

Most of the time TdP is self-limiting and only produces transient syncope but it can also degenerate into VF leading to cardiac arrest.

Diagnosis

Per the 2009 AHA/ACCF/HRS guidelines,[15] the QT interval should be measured in the lead with longest QT (typically lead V2 or V3) and QTc cutoffs for adults are 460 milliseconds or greater for women and 450 milliseconds or greater for men. A QTc greater than 500 milliseconds is considered high risk for TdP. There is no consensus recommendation for which formula should be used to calculate the QTc but the Bazett formula ($QTc = QT/\sqrt{RR}$) is frequently used. In general, QT interval determination should be avoided in the presence of tachycardia or bradycardia. It is also recommended to obtain serial ECGs and manually validate the computer-generated QTc intervals.

The diagnosis of congenital LQTS is made by genetic testing. Not every patient with a prolonged QTc interval warrants this testing, so the LQTS Diagnostic Criteria (**Table 2**) are commonly used for risk stratification.

Management

The acute management of patients with LQTS, congenital or acquired, presenting with TdP includes unsynchronized cardioversion as needed, administration of intravenous magnesium, correction of hypokalemia if present, and removal of any QT prolonging drugs. Electrical overdrive pacing can be used for cases refractory to pharmacologic treatment. Chemical overdrive pacing, typically with isoproterenol, can be used for patients with known acquired LQTS. Congenital LQTS is considered adrenergic dependent and patients will often be on beta-blockers such as propranolol or nadolol for dysrhythmia prevention, so the use of a beta-agonist such as isoproterenol is

---

Box 2
Noncongenital causes of a prolonged QTc interval

- Cardiac ischemia
- Elevated intracranial pressure
- Hypocalcemia
- Hypokalemia
- Hypomagnesemia
- Hypothermia
- Medications

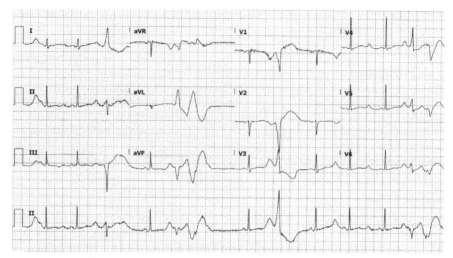

Fig. 5. ECG of a patient with long QT syndrome with frequent R-on-T PVCs that can trigger torsades de pointes. (*Courtesy of* Jeremy G. Berberian, MD.)

contraindicated. Long-term treatments include oral beta-blockers, left cardiac sympathetic denervation, and placement of an implantable cardiac defibrillator. For patients who are asymptomatic and identified incidentally, disposition should be made in consultation with a cardiologist because the first manifestation of LQTS can be SCD.

Table 2
LQTS diagnostic criteria[16]

	Findings		Points
ECG (In the absence of medications or disorders known to affect these ECG features)	QTc (= QT/√RR)	≥480 ms	3
		460–479 ms	2
		450–459 ms (in men)	1
		≥480 ms during fourth minute of recovery from exercise stress test	1
	Torsade de pointes[a]		2
	T wave alternans		1
	Notched T wave in 3 leads		1
	Low heart rate for age (or less than second percentile for age)		0.5
Clinical history	Syncope[a]	W/stress	2
		W/o stress	1
Family history	Family member(s) w/definite LQTS[b]		1
	Unexplained SCD at age younger than 30 years in immediate family[b]		0.5
	[a]Mutually exclusive [b]The same family member cannot be counted for both criteria		
	Scoring: • ≤1.0 point = low probability of LQTS • 1.5–3.0 points = intermediate probability of LQTS • ≥3.5 points = high probability of LQTS		

[a] Mutually exclusive.
[b] The same family member cannot be counted for both criteria.

DISCLOSURE

The author has nothing to disclose.

REFERENCES

1. Zipes DP, Wellens HJ. Sudden cardiac death. Circulation 1998;98(21):2334–51. PMID: 9826323.
2. Diez D, Brugada J. Diagnosis and management of arrhythmogenic right ventricular dysplasia: an article from the e-journal of the esc council for cardiology practice. European Society of Cardiology; 2008.
3. McKenna WJ, Thiene G, Nava A, et al. Diagnosis of arrhythmogenic right ventricular dysplasia/cardiomyopathy. task force of the working group myocardial and pericardial disease of the european society of cardiology and of the scientific council on cardiomyopathies of the international society and federation of cardiology. Br Heart J 1994;71(3):215–8. PMID: 8142187; PMCID: PMC483655.
4. Marcus FI, McKenna WJ, Sherrill D, et al. Diagnosis of arrhythmogenic right ventricular cardiomyopathy/dysplasia: proposed modification of the Task Force Criteria. Eur Heart J 2010;31(7):806–14. https://doi.org/10.1093/eurheartj/ehq025. Epub 2010 Feb 19. PMID: 20172912; PMCID: PMC2848326.
5. Wang J, Yang B, Chen H, et al. Epsilon waves detected by various electrocardiographic recording methods: In patients with arrhythmogenic right ventricular cardiomyopathy. Tex Heart Inst J 2010;37(4):405–11.
6. Catalano O, Antonaci S, Moro G, et al. Magnetic resonance investigations in Brugada syndrome reveal unexpectedly high rate of structural abnormalities. Eur Heart J 2009;30:2241–8.
7. Quan XQ, Li S, Liu R, et al. A meta-analytic review of prevalence for Brugada ECG patterns and the risk for death. Medicine 2016;95:e5643.
8. Takigawa M, Noda T, Shimizu W, et al. Seasonal and circadian distributions of ventricular fibrillation in patients with Brugada syndrome. Heart Rhythm 2008;5: 1523–7.
9. Proposed diagnostic criteria for the brugada syndrome consensus report. Circulation 2002;106(Issue 19):2514–9.
10. Juan Sieira, Brugada Pedro. The definition of the Brugada syndrome. Eur Heart J 2017;38(Issue 40):3029–34.
11. Mizusawa Y, Wilde AA. Brugada syndrome. Circ Arrhythm Electrophysiol 2012; 5(3):606–16. https://doi.org/10.1161/CIRCEP.111.964577. PMID: 22715240.
12. Ommen SR, Mital S, Burke MA, et al. 2020 AHA/ACC guideline for the diagnosis and treatment of patients with hypertrophic cardiomyopathy: a report of the American College of Cardiology/American Heart Association Joint Committee on Clinical Practice Guidelines. Circulation 2020;142:e558–631. https://doi.org/10.1161/CIR.0000000000000937.
13. Kelly BS, Mattu A, Brady WJ. Hypertrophic cardiomyopathy: electrocardiographic manifestations and other important considerations for the emergency physician. Am J Emerg Med 2007;25:72–9.
14. Schwartz PJ, Crotti L, Insolia R. Long-QT syndrome: from genetics to management. Circ Arrhythm Electrophysiol 2012;5(4):868–77. Erratum in: Circ Arrhythm Electrophysiol. 2012 Dec;5(6):e119-877. PMID: 22895603; PMCID: PMC3461497.
15. Rautaharju PM, Surawicz B, Gettes LS. AHA/ACCF/HRS recommendations for the standardization and interpretation of the electrocardiogram, part IV: the ST segment, T and U waves, and the QT interval: a scientific statement

from the American Heart Association Electrocardiography and Arrhythmias Committee, Council on Clinical Cardiology; the American College of Cardiology Foundation; and the Heart Rhythm Society. Circulation 2009;119: e241-50.

16. Schwartz PJ, Crotti L. QTc behavior during exercise and genetic testing for the long-QT syndrome. Circulation 2011;124(20):2181-4. PMID: 22083145.

The Ischemic Electrocardiogram

Daniel L. Kreider, MD*

KEYWORDS

- Ischemic • Electrocardiogram • STEMI • Myocardial infarction

KEY POINTS

- The electrocardiogram (EKG) is a rapid diagnostic test that when interpreted correctly can appropriately direct patient care.
- Myocardial ischemia manifests as various patterns on the EKG, not always within the classic ST-segment elevation myocardial infarction (STEMI) criteria.
- Not all ST-segment elevation seen on the EKG represents ischemia.
- Clinicians must recognize EKG signs of ischemia to appropriately manage acute coronary syndrome and improve patient outcomes.

INTRODUCTION

Electrocardiogram (EKG) utility ranges from the emergent diagnosis of myocardial ischemia or life-threatening arrhythmias to the routine evaluation of a pacemaker or identification of cardiac strain from longstanding hypertension. Clinicians of various medical specialties must be comfortable obtaining and interpreting an EKG as it is a vital diagnostic tool in evaluating medical patients. The EKG has a crucial role in helping clinicians recognize ischemia in patients presenting with acute coronary syndrome.[1] It is important to recognize coronary ischemia in a timely manner to help facilitate rapid treatment and coronary reperfusion if indicated. The American Heart Association (AHA)/American College of Cardiology (ACC) guidelines recommend obtaining and correctly interpreting an EKG within 10 min of arrival in all patients with suspected myocardial infarction (MI).[2]

PREVALENCE/INCIDENCE

Acute coronary syndrome is extremely prevalent in today's patient population, and clinicians frequently evaluate patients for cardiac ischemia. The differential diagnosis of chest pain ranges from a benign muscular strain to life-threatening coronary occlusion

Department of Emergency Medicine, Wellspan York Hospital, 1001 South George Street, York, PA 17403, USA
* Corresponding author.
E-mail address: Dkreider3@wellspan.org

Emerg Med Clin N Am 40 (2022) 663–678
https://doi.org/10.1016/j.emc.2022.06.006
0733-8627/22/© 2022 Elsevier Inc. All rights reserved.

requiring emergent revascularization. Chest pain accounted for greater than 5% of all emergency department visits in 2018 according to data from the National Center for Health Statistics.[3]

ACUTE CORONARY SYNDROME PATHOPHYSIOLOGY

Myocardial ischemia and infarction typically occur from coronary atherosclerosis and plaque formation with subsequent thrombosis or coronary spasm. Rupture of an unstable plaque in a coronary vessel may lead to total arterial occlusion, myocardial ischemia, and without intervention, myocardial necrosis. With prolonged ischemia, cellular metabolism is altered resulting in myocyte infarction and death. Cardiac myocytes can tolerate a certain duration of ischemia through anaerobic metabolism before infarction and subsequent necrosis becomes irreversible. Earlier reperfusion portends improved myocyte recovery and cardiac function, so time is myocardium. Although ischemia and infarction can be detected by serologic testing, the EKG permits even earlier recognition of ischemia.[4]

ELECTROCARDIOGRAPHIC INDICATORS OF ISCHEMIA

Myocardial ischemia manifests on EKG during ventricular repolarization with changes in the ST-segment and T wave. The ST-segment correlates to phase 2 of the cardiac action potential (the plateau phase), representing early ventricular repolarization. As the membrane potential does not change during this segment, the ST-segment will be isoelectric on a normal EKG. During ischemia, myocardial cell membrane potentials change in a regional pattern causing displacement of the ST-segment.[5] The J-point, or junction between the terminal QRS and initiation of the ST-segment, should be used to measure ST-segment deviation. Displacement should be measured from the isoelectric TP-segment in patients with a stable baseline. Otherwise, the onset of the QRS complex should be used[6] (**Fig. 1**). The T wave correlates to phase 3 of the cardiac action potential (the rapid phase), representing rapid ventricular repolarization. The T

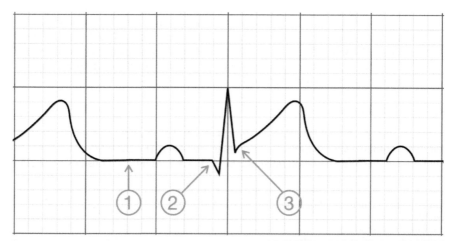

Fig. 1. ST-segment elevation: Measure ST elevation using the TP-segment (*arrow* 1) or QRS onset (*arrow* 2) as a reference point. ST elevation should be measured to the ST-segment onset or J-point (*arrow* 3). Using the top of the EKG line tracing, the measured difference is the scale of ST-segment elevation.

wave is typically concordant with the polarity of the QRS complex and may become enlarged, flattened, or inverted in the presence of ischemia.[5]

Ventricular Ischemia–Non-ST-segment elevation myocardial infarction (NSTEMI)

Subendocardial ischemia can manifest on the EKG as ST-segment depressions and/ or T-wave inversions (**Box 1**).[5] Transient ST-segment changes at rest with symptoms are also suggestive of ischemia.[7] ST-segment depression in patients presenting with acute coronary syndrome (ACS) suggests a worse prognosis and higher mortality rate.[8] The scale of ST-segment depression (ie, the total number of leads and the magnitude of depth) was found to correlate with the degree of ischemia and prognosis.[8] The prognostic value of T-wave inversions is less clear, but there is evidence that the presence of T-wave inversions in $\geq$5–6 leads is predictive of adverse outcomes.[8]

Ventricular Ischemia–STEMI

Transmural cardiac ischemia manifests electrocardiographically as ST-segment elevation and identifies a patient population that requires emergent coronary reperfusion. ST-segment elevation is localized regionally by the affected EKG leads.[5] Greater ischemia causes increased ST-segment elevation and involves more EKG leads.[6] ST-segment depressions manifest in leads opposite the vector producing elevation, termed reciprocal changes. Note that reciprocal ST-depressions support, but are not required for, the diagnosis of STEMI. Early recognition of STEMI has been shown to improve patient outcomes.[2] See **Box 2** for electrocardiographic criteria suggestive of myocardial ischemia with STEMI, and **Box 3** for criteria using supplemental EKG leads.[6]

Electrocardiographically Silent Myocardial Infarction

A silent or unrecognized MI is also a consideration in an asymptomatic patient with specific EKG changes without a recent ACS or revascularization event. Risk factors include older age, male, diabetes, insulin dependence, chronic kidney disease, and previous cardiovascular disease. These events are important to recognize as they make up a large percentage of nonfatal MIs and contribute to increased mortality.[9,10] Several nonischemic conditions may also demonstrate associated Q waves: preexcitation, cardiomyopathy, cardiac amyloidosis, left bundle branch block (LBBB), myocardial hypertrophy, myocarditis, acute cor pulmonale, hyperkalemia. Silent MIs can be identified using serial EKGs, historical evidence of ACS, and additional imaging modalities. Prior EKGs are helpful in differentiating acute and chronic events.[6] See **Box 4** for electrocardiographic criteria suggestive of prior MI without identifiable nonischemic causes.

Additional Ischemic Findings

Myocardial ischemia on EKG is a dynamic process, with a progression from hyperacute T waves to T-wave inversions and Q waves following the completion of an

---

Box 1
AHA/ACC EKG findings suggestive of myocardial ischemia in the absence of BBB or left ventricular hypertrophy (LVH)[6]

NSTEMI Criteria

New ST-depression $\geq$0.5 mm in two contiguous leads

New T-wave inversion $\geq$1.0 mm in two contiguous leads with prominent R wave or R/S ratio >1

Box 2
AHA/ACC criteria for myocardial ischemia in the absence of BBB or LVH.[6]

New, or presumed new, ST-segment elevation (STE) at the J-point in ≥ 2 anatomically contiguous leads

≥ 1.0 mm STE in all leads other than V_2–V_3

≥ 2.5 mm STE in V_2–V_3 in men <40

≥ 2.0 mm STE in V_2–V_3 in men ≥ 40

≥ 1.5 mm STE in V_2–V_3 in women of all ages

Increase of ≥ 1.0 mm STE in V_2–V_3 when compared with previous EKG

---

infarct[4] (**Fig. 2**). In patients with persistent symptoms, consider serial EKGs at 15–30-min intervals.[6] Dynamic EKG changes that transiently appear during a symptomatic episode may imply underlying ischemia and severe occlusive coronary disease. Additional considerations for identifying patients at high risk to develop adverse cardiac outcomes include: ongoing ischemic chest pain, heart failure, hemodynamic instability, previous cardiac history, and elevated cardiac biomarkers.[11] Arrhythmias, bundle branch blocks, conduction delays, and poor R-wave progression may also suggest myocardial ischemia.[7]

STEMI EQUIVALENTS

Not all electrocardiographic findings that suggest coronary occlusion and ischemia fall within the outlined STEMI criteria. Several additional EKG patterns, termed STEMI equivalents, may suggest coronary occlusion in need of more aggressive therapy and consideration of percutaneous coronary intervention (PCI).[13]

de Winter T-Waves

RJ de Winter published a case series in the *NEJM* describing a new pattern of ischemia without the classic ST-segment elevation associated with coronary occlusion.[14] EKG evidence of ST-segment depressions ≥ 1 mm in precordial leads (V_1–V_6) with associated tall, positive, symmetric T-waves suggests the de Winter pattern (**Fig. 3**). This pattern is often accompanied by 0.5–1 mm of ST-segment elevation in lead aVR. Found in approximately 2% of angiographically confirmed anterior MIs, de Winter pattern is associated with LAD occlusion. These findings were observed in the setting of normal potassium levels without significant QRS widening.[14] This pattern is persistent and should be differentiated from other causes of transient peaked T waves. These electrocardiographic findings in a patient presenting with ischemic chest pain are highly predictive of acute LAD occlusion, and this patient population should be considered for immediate revascularization.[15–17]

Box 3
AHA/ACC criteria for myocardial ischemia using supplemental leads[6]

Supplemental Lead Criteria

≥ 0.5 mm STE (≥ 1.0 mm in men <40 years) in ≥ 1 posterior leads V_7–V_9

≥ 0.5 mm STE (≥ 1.0 mm STE in men <30 years) in V_3R and/or V_4R

Box 4
AHA/ACC EKG criteria for myocardial ischemia in the absence of LBBB or LVH.[6]

Silent MI Criteria (in the absence on nonischemic causes)

Q wave > 20 ms or QS complex in V_2–V_3

Q wave $\geq$30 ms and $\geq$ 1 mm deep or QS complex in either I and aVL, II and aVF, or V_4–V_6

R wave >40 ms in V_1–V_2 and R/S > 1 with positive concordant T wave

---

Wellens Syndrome

Wellens syndrome, also called "LAD coronary T-wave syndrome," was first described in 1982 by Dutch cardiologist Dr. Hein J.J. Wellens.[18] These electrocardiographic findings depict a reperfusion pattern from a proximal LAD stenosis/lesion seen in a pain free state with recent anginal symptoms. The diagnostic findings include[19,20]

- Biphasic (type A) or deeply inverted (type B) T waves in the mid-precordial leads, typically V2–V3 (**Fig. 4**)
- Isoelectric or minimal (<1 mm) ST-segment elevation
- No precordial Q waves
- Preserved precordial R-wave progression
- Normal or minimally elevated troponins

Biphasic (positive then negative) T-waves, called Wellens type A, are an early finding, whereas deeply inverted T-waves, called Wellens type B, are a later finding and more common. These EKG findings can persist for weeks as they do not resolve until the LAD lesion is treated. Coronary angiography is required to evaluate the need for early angioplasty or coronary bypass surgery,[21] and provocative testing, especially exercise stress testing, should be avoided as it could precipitate an acute MI or cardiac arrest. A large percentage of patients presenting with this syndrome have been shown to develop an extensive anterior wall infarction, highlighting the importance of accurate recognition, urgent angiography, and subsequent reperfusion therapy.[18]

Posterior Myocardial Infarction

Isolated posterior MIs are difficult to diagnose due to the subtle electrocardiographic findings. Infarction of the posterior myocardium has been described as occurring in 15% to 21% of all acute MIs, most often with a concurrent inferior or lateral MI, of which 3% to 5% are isolated posterior MIs diagnosed by posterior leads.[22] The posterior descending artery (PDA) is supplied by the right coronary artery (RCA) in 70% of the population (right dominant circulation), left circumflex artery (LCx) in 10% of the population (left dominant circulation), and the remaining 20% of the population are supplied by both vessels (codominant circulation). Owing to coronary anatomy, the majority of posterior MIs involves the RCA and may be associated with arrhythmias in the setting of ischemic nodal involvement.

Progression of T-waves in MI

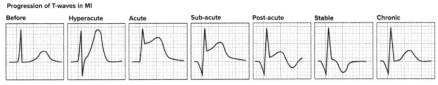

Before   Hyperacute   Acute   Sub-acute   Post-acute   Stable   Chronic

Fig. 2. Progression of T-waves in MI. (*From* Berberian JG, et al. EMRA EKG Guide. Irving: EMRA; 2017. p.6; with permission.[12])

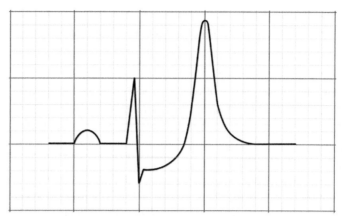

Fig. 3. de Winter T waves: Precordial leads demonstrating upsloping ST-segment depressions with tall symmetric T waves.

ST-segment elevation may accompany a posterior MI with involvement of the inferior or lateral coronary distribution.[23] However, isolated posterior circulation occlusion is indirectly observed through the EKG as ST-segment depressions in the anterior precordial leads. The anteroseptal leads are directed toward the internal surface of the posterior myocardium, and because the electrical activity is recorded from the anterior side of the heart, the typical injury pattern of ST elevation and Q waves becomes inverted. The anterior ST-segment depressions of a posterior MI represent reciprocal changes to the ST-segment elevation of the posterior myocardium. EKG findings include ST-segment depressions $\geq$0.5 mm in leads V_1–V_3, upright T waves, and tall R waves in V_1–V_2 (**Fig. 5**). These findings are in contrast to the ST-segment elevation, inverted T waves, and deep Q waves of the posterior EKG, respectively.[24]

On the 12-lead EKG, no leads directly observe the posterior myocardium. Posterior wall ischemia may be electrically silent with a normal EKG.[2] With high clinical suspicion for ACS in the setting of a nondiagnostic EKG, it is reasonable to obtain a posterior EKG with leads V_7–V_9 on the posterior chest wall to evaluate for isolated posterior circulation occlusion. Inferobasal or posterior infarction can be diagnosed in leads V_7–V_9 with $\geq$0.5 mm ST-segment elevation ($\geq$1.0 mm ST-segment elevation in men <40 years) in any one lead.[6]

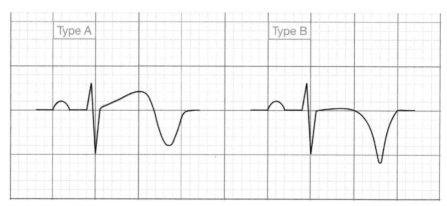

Fig. 4. Wellens Pattern: Precordial leads demonstrating biphasic (Type A) or deeply inverted T waves (Type B).

Right Ventricular Myocardial Infarction

Right ventricular infarction is rare in isolation but associated with up to half of inferior wall MIs.[25] Right ventricular myocardial infarction (RVMI) usually occurs via proximal RCA occlusion and can lead to right ventricle (RV) dilation, decreased contractility, and ventricular dysrhythmias causing a loss of cardiac output and development of cardiogenic shock. Right atrium (RA) involvement may further complicate RV dysfunction through atrial tachydysrhythmias, bradydysrhythmias, and AV blocks.[26] Atrioventricular (AV) dyssynchrony has been shown to cause lower cardiac output requiring increased ionotropic support and earlier revascularization.[27]

When treating patients with confirmed or suspected RVMI, it is critical to avoid hypotension by optimizing preload with intravenous (IV) fluids and avoiding vasodilatory medications. It is also important to treat dysrhythmias, especially those that lead to atrioventricular dyssynchrony and decreased cardiac output.[28] Owing to the hemodynamic and arrhythmogenic complications, RV involvement is associated with an increase in short-term morbidity and mortality when compared with isolated inferior infarction. Early revascularization by PCI leads to improved mortality. The increased complications and unique management of RV infarction requires prompt identification and treatment.[28,29]

The right heart is not well visualized on the standard 12-lead EKG, but findings suggestive of an RVMI include ST-segment elevations in leads V_1 and aVR, ST-segment elevations in lead III > lead II, or reciprocal ST-segment depressions in leads I and aVL (**Fig. 6**). When suspecting RV involvement, consider obtaining right-sided EKG leads by mirroring the standard 12-lead EKG arrangement on the right chest.[2,28] Diagnostic criteria for RVMI include $\geq$0.5 mm STE in V_3R–V_4R ($\geq$1.0 mm STE in men <30 years). Reciprocal ST-segment depression in aVL exhibits high sensitivity and specificity for identification of RVMI.[30,31] It is important to note that lack of ST-segment elevation on right-sided leads does not exclude RVMI and additional cardiac imaging may be helpful.[6]

ST Elevation in Lead aVR with Diffuse ST Depressions

The clinical significance of the pattern of ST-segment elevation in lead aVR ± lead V1 with diffuse ST-segment depressions (**Fig. 7**) is controversial because of its broad differential diagnosis that includes both ACS and non-ACS causes. One study found less

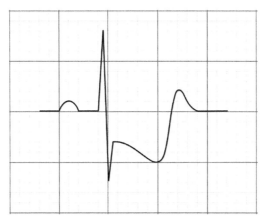

Fig. 5. Posterior MI: Pattern seen in anterior precordial leads demonstrating tall R waves, ST-segment depressions, and upright T waves.

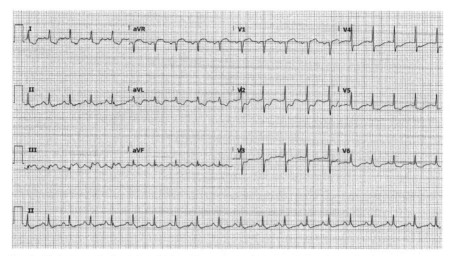

Fig. 6. Right Ventricular MI: Inferior ST-segment elevation in lead III > lead II, ST-segment elevations in leads V1 and aVR, and ST-segment depressions in leads I and aVL (image courtesy of Jeremy Berberian, MD).

than one-third of patients presenting with this EKG pattern had MI, emphasizing the broad differential diagnosis of circumferential subendocardial ischemia.[32] The 2018 Fourth Universal Definition of MI acknowledges that this EKG pattern can be suggestive of multivessel disease or left main coronary artery disease but does not provide specific management recommendations.[6]

When associated with ACS, ST-segment elevation in lead aVR has important prognostic implications. Wong and colleagues[33] demonstrated an increased 30-day mortality when ≥1 mm aVR ST-segment elevation was present with anterior and inferior MIs.[34] In ACS presentations, ST-segment elevation in lead aVR ± lead V1 with diffuse ST-segment depressions is highly suggestive of left main coronary artery (LMCA) insufficiency, proximal left anterior descending artery (LAD) insufficiency, or triple vessel disease and warrants consideration for immediate angiography.[6]

It is essential that the broad differential diagnosis for non-ACS causes is also considered, including global cardiac ischemia (eg, anemia), hypovolemic shock, tachydysrhythmias, pulmonary embolism, electrolyte abnormalities, and aortic pathologies.[6]

T-Wave Inversion in Lead aVL

An isolated T-wave inversion in aVL may represent a subtle potential indicator of an impending inferior MI in the appropriate clinical scenario. Lead aVL is the only lead with a vector opposite that of the inferior leads, and the reciprocal changes seen in lead aVL (ie, T-wave inversion and ST-segment depression) are commonly present in inferior MIs (**Fig. 8**). In a review of admission EKGs in patients with acute inferior MIs, ST depression in lead aVL was the only initial finding of the inferior ischemia in some cases.[35] In the setting of an inferior MI, ST-segment depression in lead aVL was also found to be a sensitive and specific finding suggesting right ventricular involvement.[30,31] T-wave inversions in lead aVL have also been described in mid-LAD occlusion.[36] In a patient with ischemic chest pain, identification of reciprocal changes in lead aVL can promote early recognition of a developing inferior MI.[36]

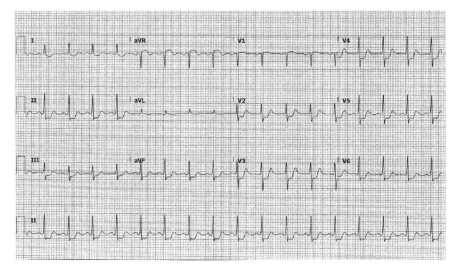

Fig. 7. Lead aVR STE: ST-segment elevation in aVR with diffuse ST-segment depressions noted throughout inferior and lateral leads (image courtesy of Jeremy Berberian, MD).

Hyperacute T-waves

There is no universal definition of hyperacute T-waves, but they are typically described as tall, broad based, symmetrical, with amplitude potentially larger than the associated QRS complex (**Fig. 9**).[37] Hyperacute T-waves can be an early EKG finding in an ischemic event, preceding ST-segment elevations and/or depressions, and the 2018 AHA/ACC guidelines recognize hyperacute T-waves in two contiguous leads

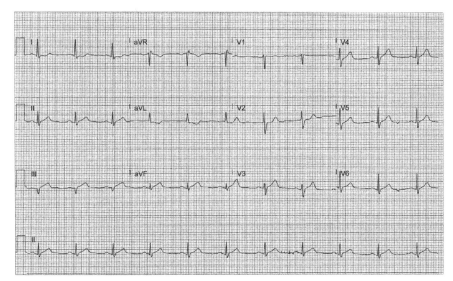

Fig. 8. Lead aVL: ST-segment depression and T-wave inversion of lead aVL with hyperacute T waves in leads II, III, aVF demonstrate a developing inferior MI (image courtesy of Jeremy Berberian, MD).

as an early sign of myocardial ischemia.[6] The significance of upright T waves as a marker of CAD was initially described in 1966 with the observation that tall and upright T-waves in the precordial leads were the earliest electrocardiographic signs of an acute MI.[38] In addition, it has been suggested that an upright T-wave in lead V_1 is associated with a higher likelihood of CAD,[39] correlated with disease of the left circumflex (LCx) artery on catheterization,[40] and is in the absence of an LBBB or LVH, a new, large upright T wave in V1 is suggestive of ischemia. The term "loss of precordial T-wave balance" is used when the T-wave amplitude in lead $V_1 > V_6$.[41]

Other causes of large T waves include hyperkalemia, LVH strain pattern, LBBB, and myopericarditis.[37] In a patient with ischemic chest pain and hyperacute T waves, management should include ACS management with serial EKGs and consideration of cardiology consultation.[37]

RECOGNIZING ISCHEMIA IN LEFT BUNDLE BRANCH BLOCK

Identifying electrocardiographic evidence to accurately diagnose STEMI in LBBB is a challenge due to the characteristic repolarization changes in asymptomatic patients. In the past, the AHA/ACC recommended emergent PCI in patients with suspected MI and a new or presumed new LBBB based on Class A evidence.[42] More recently, additional data have shown that in patients presenting with chest pain, only 13% with an LBBB had an acute MI and a new LBBB was only 42% sensitive and 65% specific for an acute MI.[43] Additional study demonstrated a 7.3% rate of biomarker-confirmed MI in patients with a new LBBB. This percentage did not significantly differ from the rate of MI in patients with a preexisting LBBB (5.2%) or patients without an LBBB (6.1%).[44] Despite the ability of an LBBB to mask ischemia, it is not specific for myocardial ischemia and using new or presumed new LBBB as an STEMI criterion results in unnecessary invasive catheterization.[42,43] Accordingly, current AHA/ACC guidelines recommend that a new or presumed new LBBB "should not be considered diagnostic of acute myocardial infarction in isolation." [45]

European guidelines for management of acute MI also recognize that a new LBBB does not necessarily predict myocardial ischemia but recommend that patients with an LBBB and clinical suspicion of ongoing ischemia "be managed in a way similar to STEMI patients, regardless of whether the LBBB is previously known." [46]

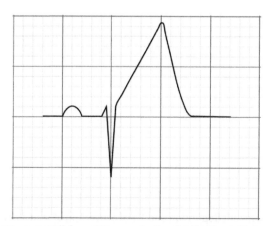

Fig. 9. Hyperacute T waves: Tall, broad T-waves in the distribution of ischemia may signify an impending MI.

Table 1 Sgarbossa criteria for MI in LBBB[47]	
Sgarbossa Criteria in Presence of LBBB	
Concordant ST elevation $\geq$1 mm in 1 or more leads	Score 5
Concordant ST depression $\geq$1 mm in lead V_1, V_2, or V_3	Score 3
Discordant ST elevation $\geq$5 mm in 1 or more leads	Score 2

Sgarbossa and colleagues proposed criteria for diagnosis of STEMI in LBBB using concordance or excessive discordance of the ST-segment and QRS as outlined by the criteria in **Table 1** and **Fig. 10**. Concordance and discordance refer to the ST-segment with respect to QRS polarity. Based on the outlined criteria, index scores $\geq$ 3 had a 36% sensitivity and 96% specificity for MI. Of note, although sensitivity was lacking, concordant ST deviation is specific for MI while excessive discordance has a moderate–high likelihood of MI.[47]

Smith and colleagues sought to improve these criteria by replacing the fixed cutoff of 5 mm for discordant ST elevation with absolute value of the ratio of ST-segment elevation to S-wave depth. This new criterion is met when the |ST/S ratio| is $\geq$ 0.25 with ST elevation $\geq$1 mm and discordant to the QRS. This modified Sgarbossa criterion was unweighted (all three rules apply) and found to have 91% sensitivity and 90% specificity.[48] The Modified Sgarbossa criteria are not mandated in the current AHA/JCC STEMI guidelines.

In 2020, Dimarco again modified the same unweighted criteria. The second rule was expanded to include concordant ST-segment depression $\geq$1 mm in any lead, improving sensitivity without compromising specificity. The third rule was replaced with discordant ST-segment deviation $\geq$1 mm with a dominant QRS complex $\leq$6 mm. This dominant complex (R|S) was defined as "the R wave in leads with a predominantly positive QRS and the Q or S wave in leads with a predominantly negative QRS, measured with respect to QRS onset." The third criteria capitalize on the association of MIs with lower QRS amplitude, producing more leads with maximum (R|S) amplitude $\leq$6 mm. These changes create the Barcelona algorithm, outlined in **Box 5** and **Fig. 11**, used to diagnose acute MIs in LBBB with 93% sensitivity and 94% specificity.[49] The Barcelona algorithm is not mandated in the current AHA/ACC STEMI guidelines.

Complications exist with both over and underdiagnosing the need for emergent reperfusion in patients with LBBB. While awaiting external validation, these new criteria may prove to be a great addition in the challenging evaluation for ischemia

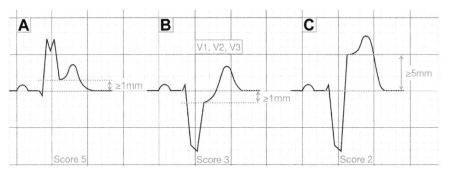

Fig. 10. Sgarbossa Criteria depicted visually. Examples of concordant ST-segment elevation (A), concordant ST-segment depression (B), and discordant ST-segment elevation (C).

Box 5
Barcelona algorithm for MI in LBBB[49]

Barcelona algorithm in presence of LBBB

Concordant ST elevation ≥1 mm in 1 or more leads

Concordant ST depression ≥1 mm in 1 or more leads

Discordant ST deviation ≥1 mm in 1 or more leads with max (R|S) ≤6 mm

---

in LBBBs. Clinicians should consider electrocardiographic findings, hemodynamics, cardiac biomarkers, and diagnostic imaging when determining need for further diagnostic and therapeutic intervention.[49,50]

STEMI MIMICS

Clinicians must also recognize STEMI mimics or cofounders that do not represent ischemia to prevent harm from unnecessary intervention. Cardiac pathology other than coronary ischemia may contribute to similar ST-segment and T-wave abnormalities.[6] Recognizing the characteristic ST-segment changes of left ventricular hypertrophy, early repolarization, left ventricular aneurysm, Takotsubo cardiomyopathy, myopericarditis, and hyperkalemia is critical to avoid misdiagnosis and delay in definitive management. Through attentive evaluation of the subtle electrocardiographic changes of STEMI equivalents and STEMI mimics, a clinician may successfully differentiate these patterns and proceed with appropriate management.[6,51]

SUMMARY

Clinical context and EKG pattern recognition is critical as EKG changes suggestive of ischemia may vary based on the duration, severity, and distribution of myocardial ischemia. Interpreting the EKG is an essential skill for all clinicians. It is important to remember that not all ST-segment elevation requires reperfusion, and not all patients that require reperfusion manifest classic ST-segment elevations. Although the EKG does not have perfect sensitivity for coronary occlusion, one can improve early recognition by increasing familiarity with the characteristic patterns of ischemia and

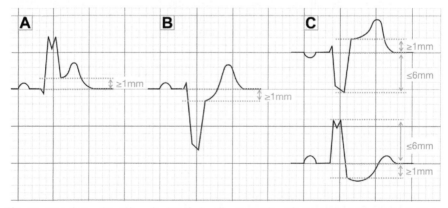

Fig. 11. Barcelona algorithm depicted visually. Examples of concordant ST-segment elevation (*A*), discordant ST-segment depression (*B*), and discordant ST-segment deviation with max (R|S) ≤6 mm (*C*).

obtaining serial EKGs. Through meticulous electrocardiographic interpretation, accurate clinical history taking, and appropriate supplemental diagnostic testing, health care providers may recognize ischemia early, provide appropriate ACS management, and improve patient care.[13]

CLINICS CARE POINTS

- AHA/ACC criteria outline ST-segment elevation required to diagnose myocardial ischemia. Posterior and right sided supplemental leads require less ST-segment elevation.
- The electrocardiographically silent MI can be recognized by a newly developed Q wave pattern and are important to recognized as they are associated with increased patient mortality.
- Myocardial ischemia is an electrocardiographically dynamic process progressing from hyperacute T waves to T wave inversions and eventual Q waves.
- One must be able to identify STEMI equivalents, as not all electrocardiographic findings suggesting coronary occlusion and ischemia fall within outlined STEMI criteria.
- Use Sgarbossa criteria and Barcelona algorithm to recognize ischemia in left bundle branch block.
- Identify STEMI mimics and consider clinical context as not all ST-segment abnormalities represent coronary ischemia.

DISCLOSURE

The author has nothing to disclose.

REFERENCES

1. Thaler MS. The only EKG book you'll ever need. Philadelphia: Lippincott Williams & Wilkins; 2012. p. 1–60.
2. Cairns C, Kang K, Santo L. National hospital ambulatory medical care survey: 2018 emergency department summary tables. Available at: https://www.cdc.gov/nchs/data/nhamcs/web_tables/2018_ed_web_tables-508.pdf.   Accessed January 10, 2022.
3. Gulati M, Levy PD, Mukherjee D, et al. 2021 AHA/ACC/ASE/CHEST/SAEM/SCCT/SCMR Guideline for the Evaluation and Diagnosis of Chest Pain. Circulation 2021; 144(22):368–454.
4. ST segment elevation in acute myocardial ischemia and differential diagnoses. In: Clinical ECG interpretation. Available at. https://ecgwaves.com/topic/myocardial-ischemia-infarction-reaction-ecg-changes-symptoms/. Accessed January 10, 2022.
5. Dubin D. Infarction. In: Rapid interpretation of EKG's. Fort Myers (FL): Cover Publishing Company; 2000. p. 259–308.
6. Thygesen K, Alpert JS, Jaffe AS, et al. Fourth universal definition of myocardial infarction. Circulation 2018;138(20):618–51.
7. Amsterdam EA, Wenger NK, Brindis RG, et al. 2014 AHA/ACC guideline for the management of patients with Non-ST-elevation acute coronary syndromes. J Am Coll Cardiol 2014;64(24):139–228.
8. Collet JP, Thiele H, Barbato E, et al. 2020 ESC Guidelines for the management of acute coronary syndromes in patients presenting without persistent ST-segment elevation. Eur Heart J 2021;42(19):1813–927.

9. Burgess DC, Hunt D, Li L, et al. Incidence and predictors of silent myocardial infarction in type 2 diabetes and the effect of fenofibrate: an analysis from the Fenofibrate Intervention and Event Lowering in Diabetes (FIELD) study. Eur Heart J 2010;31(1):92–9.

10. Liu CK, Greenspan G, Piccirillo RT. Atrial infarction of the heart. Circulation 1961; 23:331–8.

11. Braunwald E, Antman EM, Beasley JW, et al. ACC/AHA guidelines for the management of patients with unstable angina and non–st-segment elevation myocardial infarction. Circulation 2000;102(10):1193–209.

12. Berberian JG, Levine BJ, Brady WJ, et al. EMRA EKG guide. Irving: EMRA; 2017. p. 1–6.

13. Asatryan B, Vaisnora L, Manavifar N. Electrocardiographic diagnosis of life-threatening STEMI equivalents: when every minute counts. J Am Coll Cardiol Case Rep 2019;1(4):666–8.

14. de Winter RJ, Verouden NJ, Wellens HJ, et al. A new ECG sign of proximal LAD occlusion. N Engl J Med 2008;359(19):2071–3.

15. Morris NP, Body R. The De Winter ECG pattern: morphology and accuracy for diagnosing acute coronary occlusion: systematic review. J Emerg Med 2017; 24(4):236–42.

16. Zhan ZQ, Li Y, Han LH. The de winter ECG pattern: distribution and morphology of ST depression. Ann Noninvasive Electrocardiol 2020;25(5):1–9.

17. Gerson MC, Phillips JF, Morris SN. Exercise-induced U-wave inversion as a marker of stenosis of the left anterior descending coronary artery. Circulation 1979;60(5):1014–20.

18. de Zwaan C, Bär FW, Wellens HJ. Characteristic electrocardiographic pattern indicating a critical stenosis high in left anterior descending coronary artery in patients admitted because of impending myocardial infarction. Am Heart J 1982; 103:730–6.

19. Al-assaf O, Abdulghani M, Musa A, et al. Wellen's syndrome. Circulation 2019; 140(22):1851–2.

20. Rhinehardt J, Brady WJ, Perron AD, et al. Electrocardiographic manifestations of Wellens syndrome. Am J Emerg Med 2002;20(7):638–43.

21. Avram A, Chioncel V, Iancu A. Wellens sign: monography and single center experience. Maedica 2021;16(2):216–22.

22. van Gorselen EO, Verheugt FW, Meursing BT, et al. Posterior myocardial infarction: the dark side of the moon. Neth Heart J 2007;15(1):16–21.

23. Lizzo JM, Chowdhury YS. Posterior myocardial infarction. In: StatPearls. Treasure Island (FL): StatPearls Publishing; 2021. Available at: https://www.ncbi.nlm.nih.gov/books/NBK553168/.

24. Rokos IC, French WJ, Mattu A, et al. Appropriate cardiac cath lab activation: optimizing electrocardiogram interpretation and clinical decision-making for acute ST-elevation myocardial infarction. Am Heart J 2010;160(6):995–1003.

25. Goldstein JA. Right heart ischemia: pathophysiology, natural history, and clinical management. Prog Cardiovasc Dis 1998;40:325–41.

26. Jim MH, Siu CW, Chan AO, et al. Prognostic implications of PR-segment depression in inferior leads in acute inferior myocardial infarction. Clin Cardiol 2006; 29(8):363–8.

27. Goldstein JA, Barzilai B, Rosamond TL, et al. Determinants of hemodynamic compromise with severe right ventricular infarction. Circulation 1990;82(2): 359–68.

28. Haddad F, Doyle R, Murphy DJ, et al. Right ventricular function in cardiovascular disease, part II: pathophysiology, clinical importance, and management of right ventricular failure. Circulation 2008;117(13):1717–31.

29. Kakouros N, Cokkinos DV. Right ventricular myocardial infarction: pathophysiology, diagnosis, and management. Postgrad Med J 2010;86(1022):719–28.

30. Turhan H, Yilmaz MB, Yetkin E, et al. Diagnostic value of aVL derivation for right ventricular involvement in patients with acute inferior myocardial infarction. Ann Noninvasive Electrocardiol 2003;8(3):185–8.

31. Rashduni DL, Tannenbaum AK. Utility of ST segment depression in lead AVL in the diagnosis of right ventricular infarction. N J Med 2003;100(11):35–7.

32. Knotts RJ, WIlson JM, Kim E, et al. Diffuse ST depression with ST elevation in aVR: is this pattern specific for global ischemia due to the left main coronary artery disease? J Electrocardiol 2013;46(3):240–8.

33. Wong CK, Gao W, Stewart RA, et al. aVR ST elevation: an important but neglected sign in ST elevation acute myocardial infarction. Eur Heart J 2010;31:1845–53.

34. Schwaiger JP, Mair J. Left main occlusion – a classic electrocardiogram. Wien Klin Wochenschr 2016;128:521–3.

35. Birnbaum Y, Sclarovsky S, Mager A, et al. ST segment depression in aVL: A sensitive marker for acute inferior myocardial infarction. Eur Heart J 1993;14(1):4–7.

36. Hassen GW, Talebi S, Fernaine G, et al. Lead aVL on electrocardiogram: emerging as important lead in early diagnosis of myocardial infarction. Am J Emerg Med 2014;32(7):785–8.

37. Levis JT. ECG diagnosis: hyperacute T waves. Perm J 2015;19(3):79.

38. Pinto IJ, Nanda NC, Biswas AK, et al. Tall upright T waves in the precordial leads. Circulation 1967;36(5):708–16.

39. Stankovic I, Milekic K, Vlahovic Stipac A, et al. Upright T wave in precordial lead V1 indicates the presence of significant coronary artery disease in patients undergoing coronary angiography with otherwise unremarkable electrocardiogram. Herz 2012;37(7):756–61.

40. Manno BV, Hakki A, Iskandrian AS, et al. Significance of the upright T wave in precordial lead V1 in adults with coronary artery disease. J Am Coll Cardiol 1983; 1(5):1213–5.

41. Tewelde SZ, Mattu A, Brady WJ Jr. Pitfalls in electrocardiographic diagnosis of acute coronary syndrome in low-risk chest pain. West J Emerg Med 2017; 18(4):601–6.

42. Antman EM, Anbe DT, Armstrong PW, et al. ACC/AHA guidelines for the management of patients with ST-elevation myocardial infarction (committee to revise the 1999 guidelines). J Am Coll Cardiol 2004;44:671–719.

43. Kontos MC, McQueen RH, Jesse RL, et al. Can myocardial infarction be rapidly identified in emergency department patients who have left bundle-branch block? Ann Emerg Med 2001;37(5):431–8.

44. Chang AM, Shofer FS, Tabas JA, et al. Lack of association between left bundle-branch block and acute myocardial infarction in symptomatic ED patients. Am J Emerg Med 2009;27(8):916–21.

45. O'Gara PT, Kushner FG, Ascheim DD, et al. 2013 ACCF/AHA Guideline for the Management of ST-Elevation Myocardial Infarction: Executive Summary. Circulation 2013;127(4):362–425.

46. Ibanez B, James S, Agewall S, et al. 2017 ESC guidelines for the management of acute myocardial infarction in patients presenting with ST-segment elevation. Eur Heart J 2018;39:119–77.

47. Sgarbossa EB, Pinski SL, Barbagelata A, et al. Electrocardiographic diagnosis of evolving acute myocardial infarction in the presence of left bundle-branch block. N Engl J Med 1996;334:481–7.
48. Smith SW, Dodd KW, Henry TD, et al. Diagnosis of ST elevation myocardial infarction in the presence of left bundle branch block with the ST elevation to S-wave ratio in a modified Sgarbossa rule. Ann Emerg Med 2012;60:766–76.
49. Di Marco A, Rodriguez M, Cinca J, et al. New electrocardiographic algorithm for the diagnosis of acute myocardial infarction in patients with left bundle branch block. J Am Heart Assoc 2020;9(14):1–15.
50. Macfarlane PW. New ECG criteria for acute myocardial infarction in patients with left bundle branch block. J Am Heart Assoc 2020;9(14):1–5.
51. Nable JV, Lawner BJ. Chameleons: Electrocardiogram Imitators of ST- Segment Elevation Myocardial Infarction. Emerg Med Clin North Am 2015;33:529–37.

Pacemaker Malfunction– Review of Permanent Pacemakers and Malfunctions Encountered in the Emergency Department

William Brandon White, DO, Jeremy G. Berberian, MD*

KEYWORDS

- Pacemaker • Malfunction • Emergency • Magnet

KEY POINTS

- Common pacemaker modes include VOO: the ventricle is paced asynchronously, VVI: the ventricle is paced and sensed, and DDD: both the atria and ventricle are paced and sensed.
- Pacemaker malfunctions include the following:
  - Failure to sense: Pacemaker fails to sense native cardiac activity, leading to asynchronous pacing.
  - Failure to capture: Delivery of pacing stimulus without subsequent myocardial depolarization.
  - Failure to pace: Pacing stimulus is not generated when expected.
- Pacemaker-mediated tachycardia is a reentry tachycardia that is very similar to, and treated the same as, antidromic atrioventricular reentrant (or reciprocating) tachycardia (AVRT) except that the pacemaker replaces the accessory pathway.
- Cardioversion/defibrillation can be performed on patients with pacemakers. Pads should be placed 8 to 12 cm from the pulse generator in the anterior–posterior configuration and the lowest energy indicated for the dysrhythmia should be used.

INTRODUCTION

Since the first implanted pacemaker in 1958, implantable cardiac electronic devices have made tremendous strides to improve morbidity and mortality for patients with conduction disease. Furthermore, advancements in technology have allowed

Department of Emergency Medicine, Christiana Care, 4755 Ogletown Stanton Road, Newark, DE 19718, USA
* Corresponding author.
E-mail address: Jgberberian@gmail.com

Emerg Med Clin N Am 40 (2022) 679–691
https://doi.org/10.1016/j.emc.2022.06.007
0733-8627/22/© 2022 Elsevier Inc. All rights reserved.

emed.theclinics.com

pacemakers to have better longevity, functionality, and miniaturization, even to the point of leadless pacemakers.[1,2] Many of these advancements have resulted in better performance and less complications associated with pacemakers. Millions of people have received pacemaker devices in the United States[3] and less than 5% of patients develop symptomatic pacemaker malfunction after implantation.[4] Although malfunctions are occurring less commonly with developments in pacemaker technology and close follow-up with electrophysiologists, pacemaker malfunctions still occur and can be a cause of mortality.[3] Emergency department physicians should be well versed on evaluating pacemaker function and identifying malfunction when present. This discussion will focus on pacemaker malfunction. Discussion of postoperative and other complications such as thrombosis, hematoma, pericardial effusions, and infection are outside the scope of this article. To understand potential pacemaker malfunctions, it is critical to have a strong fundamental understanding of pacemaker functionality and nomenclature.

Case Challenge

A 65-year-old man presents to the emergency department complaining of palpitations. He is hemodynamically stable, and an electrocardiogram (ECG) is obtained (**Fig. 1**). Please review the ECG, and we will return to this case in a later discussion.

Components of Permanent Pacemakers

Cardiac pacemakers provide an extrinsic means to generate cardiac depolarization in patients with bradyarrhythmias and/or conduction disease to improve cardiac function. From a nuts-and-bolts perspective, the pacemaker must be equipped to perform sensing and pacing function and is composed of a pulse generator and leads (electrodes).

Pulse generators are the power source of the pacemaker and provide the pacemaker stimulus. Lithium batteries of the generator often last 4 to 10 years but can be variable depending on the requirements placed on the battery by the device and programming. Pacemakers use features that identify recommended replacement

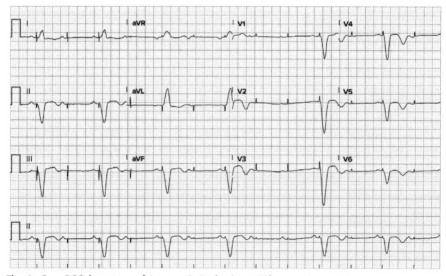

Fig. 1. Case ECG (courtesy of Jeremy G. Berberian, MD).

times as well as indicators for elective replacement. Lithium batteries also gradually decrease output overtime unlike prior batteries These features provide the patient and cardiologist with a safe time window to replace the battery for the device and thus are less likely to cause device malfunction.[4]

Pacemaker leads are transvenous projections with endocardial electrodes. These leads may be unipolar or bipolar. Unipolar configurations consist of leads with the antenna (sensing component) responsible for electrical signal detection extending the entire length from the pulse generator to the myocardium, where the electrode is at the lead-myocardial interface. This generates a larger amplitude spike on the ECG and a large antenna effect, increasing the likelihood to detect noise. Bipolar configurations are designed with both the antenna and electrode positioned within the heart. This generates a much smaller pacemaker spike and antenna effect, which allows for more precise manipulation of sensing features without sensing alternative noise/signals.[4,5] Leadless devices incorporate the sensor and pulse generator together at the myocardial interface.[1,2]Sensors on pacemakers have 2 intervals that are critical to understanding pacemaker function—a refractory and an alert period. The refractory period is initiated after a paced event is detected, rendering the sensor incapable of detecting additional stimuli that would generate an inappropriate response. The alert period follows the refractory period and represents the interval when the sensor can detect stimuli and allows the device to respond with a triggered or inhibited response (ie, delivers a pacing stimulus or not). Thus, true sensing for stimuli, as well as sensing abnormalities, can only occur during the alert period.

Pacemaker Nomenclature

Pacemaker functional coding is described using a 5-position code.[6] Commonly, the code is written with only the first 3 positions, and the fourth and fifth positions may be included for completeness (**Table 1**). If only 3 or 4 positions are used, it is assumed the other positions are not applicable. The first position indicates the chamber that is paced. The second position indicates the chamber sensed. The third position indicates the mode or response position—which dictates how the pacemaker responds to sensed stimuli. The fourth position indicates the presence or absence of a rate adaptive feature that optimizes pacing rate and pacing intervals based on measured physiologic feedback, such as minute ventilation or vibration. The fifth position specifies the location (or absence) of multisite pacing. Although this coding position is rarely ever used, it can indicate pacing in both atria or ventricles, multiple stimulation sites in a single cardiac chamber, or a combination of these locations. The fifth feature is most commonly applicable to advanced heart failure patients who have undergone cardiac resynchronization therapy with biventricular pacing.

Table 1
Pacemaker nomenclature (code)[6]

First Position Chamber Paced	Second Position Chamber Sensed	Third Position Response to Sensing	Fourth Position Programmability/Rate Modulation	Fifth Position Multisite Pacing
A—Atrial	A—Atrial	I—Inhibited	P—Simple programmable	A—Atrium
V—Ventricular	V—Ventricular	T—Triggered	M—multiprogrammable	V—Ventricle
D—Dual	D—Dual	D—Dual	C—Communicating	D—Dual
O—None	O—None	O—None	R—Rate modulation	O—None
			O—None	

Table 2
Common modes of permanent pacemakers

Code	VOO	VVI	DDD
Function	• Ventricle is paced at a set rate regardless of native cardiac activity (ie, asynchronously)	• Ventricle is paced at a set rate • Pacing is inhibited if pacer senses intrinsic ventricular activity	• Pacing is triggered or inhibited based on whether native cardiac activity is sensed • Atrial pacing is inhibited if a native atrial beat is sensed • Ventricular pacing is inhibited if a native ventricular beat is sensed • The pacer triggers a ventricular beat if it senses an atrial beat (either paced or native) and there is no intrinsic ventricular beat within a programmed amount of time
Indications	• Short-term mode used for surgery or procedures • Rarely used long term	• Chronic atrial fibrillation	• AV node block with normal SA node • AV and SA node dysfunction
Pros	• Guaranteed pacing at set rate • Removes sensing function and associated malfunction risks	• Protection from lethal bradyarrhythmia • Single lead	• Physiologic pacing • (ie, allows for native pacing)
Cons	• Lacks AV synchrony • Competes with native rhythm, increased risk for R-on-T phenomenon	• Lacks AV synchrony	• Multiple leads with advanced programming

Abbreviation: AV, atrioventricular; SA, sinoatrial.

Pacemaker Modes

Pacemakers are indicated for many reasons[7] and are generally guided by the site of conduction disease, symptoms related to a bradyarrhythmia, and the absence of a reversible cause. These factors along with many others guide pacing modality selection and programmable features. The most common pacemaker modes are described in **Tables 2**.

Single-chamber pacing (atrial or ventricular) is a single lead device that only functions in a single chamber. Ventricular (VVI, VVIR) pacing provides protection against lethal bradyarrhythmia; however, it lacks atrioventricular (AV) synchrony and can result in pacemaker syndrome (see "Other Pearls and Pitfalls" section). Ventricular single lead pacing remains the most common form of pacing today; however, dual-chamber systems are becoming more common, and data suggest patients may prefer dual-chamber systems.[8] Dual-chamber devices provide physiologic pacing and have the potential to generate 4 different rhythms—normal sinus, atrial sensed with ventricular pacing (**Fig. 2**), atrial pacing with intrinsic ventricular pacing, and sequential AV pacing.

Several pacemaker modes provide "physiologic pacing." This term refers to pacemaker activity that closely resembles normal cardiac function and preserves AV synchrony. It is notable that this form of pacing may benefit patients by improving hemodynamics with AV synchrony and preventing pacemaker syndrome[8] as well as lower incidence of atrial fibrillation and thromboembolic events.[9] Although physiologic pacing improves AV dysynchrony seen in single-chamber pacing, the negative effects from long-term right ventricular (RV) pacing are still present.

RV pacing generates ventricular dysynchrony such that the right ventricle and septum contract before the left ventricle (similar to a left bundle branch block), which can worsen heart failure morbidity and mortality.[10] RV pacing using modes and programming (such as ventricular avoidance or hysteresis) that favor intrinsic conduction are actively being incorporated to combat this issue. Similarly, biventricular pacemakers attempt to restore normal, synchronized ventricular contractions in patients with heart failure to improve outcomes and functional status.[11,12]

A common feature for dual-chamber systems is automatic mode-switching capability. Devices will sense atrial activity and ventricular pace as designed. However, should an atrial dysrhythmia occur, the pacemaker will initially pace the ventricle up to a preset upper limit pacing rate. With mode switching parameter activated, the device can transiently reprogram itself to no longer monitor the native atrial rate, such as VVI. Once the atrial rate normalizes or the dysrhythmia breaks, the device can return to its original settings.[13]

Patients are usually given a wallet card that provides details regarding their device. If a patient is unable to provide any information about their device, chest radiography can provide information regarding lead placement, function, and manufacturer.

Magnet application causes the pacemaker to temporarily eliminate sensing functions and transition to an asynchronous mode, such that a device programmed as DDD will function in DOO while the magnet is in place and return to DDD when the magnet is removed. This will be important for diagnosis and treatments for pacemaker malfunctions discussed in a later discussion. Note that placing a patient in asynchronous mode does present the risk of pacemaker stimulus being delivered during a refractory (vulnerable period) creating an R-on-T phenomenon, and potential for ventricular dysrhythmias.

PACEMAKER MALFUNCTIONS

Pacemaker malfunctions can occur anywhere within the system from the pulse generator and leads to the electrode–myocardium interface. Generally, these malfunctions are categorized as failure to sense, failure to pace, and failure to capture (**Table 3**).

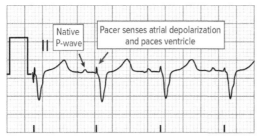

Fig. 2. Normal pacing—atrial sensed ventricular paced (ECG image courtesy of Jeremy G. Berberian, MD).

Table 3
Pacemaker malfunction synopsis

Malfunction Type	Characteristic Finding	Etiology	Management	Effect of Magnet Placement
Failure to Sense	Asynchronous pacing	1. Pulse generator failure 2. Lead failure 3. Alterations in cardiac signal 4. High or low programmed sensitivity	• Treat reversible causes • Temporary magnet placement for pacing • Cardiology consult to adjust sensitivity	Normal asynchronous pacing
Failure to Pace	Pacing stimulus is not generated when expected	1. Oversensing 2. Open circuit (ie, lead fracture) 3. Generator failure[L] (rare)	• Place magnet to identify oversensing • Temporary external pacing if unstable • Consult Cardiology for device interrogation	1. Normal asynchronous pacing 2 and 3. No pacing
Failure to Capture	Appropriate pacing stimulus without subsequent myocardial depolarization	1. Battery depletion[L] 2. Low output programming 3. Lead dislodgment[E] 4. Lead failure[L] 5. Increased capture threshold	• Treat reversible causes • Temporary external pacing if unstable • Consult Cardiology for device interrogation	Asynchronous pacing stimulus without capture

Abbreviations: E, early cause of pacemaker malfunction; L, late complication of pacemaker malfunction.

Failure to Sense–Undersensing and Oversensing

Pacemakers require monitoring of the native cardiac electrical activity to identify whether the patient's intrinsic conduction system is working appropriately or when it is inadequate. Failure to sense is used to describe when a pacemaker undersenses or oversenses, leading to asynchronous pacing or inappropriate inhibition, respectively.

Undersensing is the inability of the device to detect a native atrial or ventricular depolarization during the alert period leading to asynchronous pacing. The ECG will often show a pacer spike during or after the P-wave or QRS complex. In **Fig. 3**, the atrial pacing spike preceding the third QRS complex occurs after the atria has already started to depolarize. The pacemaker should have sensed the native atrial depolarization and inhibited atrial pacing.

Undersensing can be caused by any component of the pacemaker as well as changes in the patient's native cardiac signals.[4] Pulse generator and lead failures can lead to a signal insufficient to be detected leading to undersensing. Alternatively, the device may be programmed to an inappropriate parameter leading to poor sensitivity. Other changes such as lead maturation (myocardial changes at the implantation device due to inflammation) can lead to signals being insufficient to reach the sensitivity threshold, leading to undersensing. Finally, changes to the patient's intrinsic cardiac depolarization signal from metabolic derangements (ie, hyperkalemia[14]) or myocardial pathologic conditions (ie, cardiomyopathy, infarction) can alter the input stimulus failing to meet the sensing threshold.

Evaluating for reversible causes with medication history, ECG, and metabolic panel can identify changes to the intrinsic conduction system. Usually, undersensing can be managed by the cardiologist by adjusting the devices sensitivity parameters to allow for the detection of lower amplitude intrinsic cardiac depolarization signals.

Oversensing is characterized by the device sensing a stimulus during the alert period that is mistaken for an intrinsic depolarization. Oversensing can be a serious problem as pacemaker perception of a noncardiac signal as electrical activity will lead to inappropriate inhibition of pacing and is often misinterpreted as failure to pace. Pacemaker oversensing is due to a higher sensitivity setting, allowing the pacemaker to detect smaller signals that are falsely interpreted as myocardial depolarization. This can be a misinterpretation of cardiac signal (eg, large T-waves) or noncardiac signals such as pectoral muscle myopotentials or external electrical interference. The possibility of oversensing with electrical stimuli such as cautery is the rationale for cardiology transitioning patients with sensing features activated to asynchronous mode before surgery.

Failure to Capture

Typical pacemaker ECG is characterized by pacemaker spike, followed by cardiac depolarization. Failure to capture describes the delivery of a pacing stimulus without

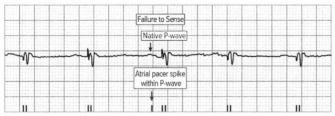

Fig. 3. Failure to sense in the atrial pacing spike preceding the third RS complex (ECG image courtesy of Jeremy G. Berberian, MD).

subsequent myocardial depolarization, as seen in **Fig. 4**. Failure to capture may be due to a variety of problems, both functional and nonfunctional. If a pacemaker-mediated impulse is delivered to the myocardium during a refractory period, the myocardium is incapable of redepolarizing, and therefore, an evoked potential will not be generated. This is an expected normal failure of the impulse not capturing and is more indicative of undersensing. Nonfunctional failure to capture can be caused by failure with the generator, the lead, or the electrode–myocardial interface.[15,16]

Failure to capture that occurs after recent pacemaker placement is commonly due to lead dislodgment or malpositioning. Frequently, this can be identified by changes in depolarization morphology of the QRS complexes when compared with old ECGs or lead placement changes noted on chest radiography. Later causes (ie, years after pacemaker placement) of failure to capture include lead failure and generator battery depletion. Chest radiography may help identify lead fractures but will not be able to identify failure of lead insulation.

An increased capture threshold can also generate loss of capture and may occur early or late after pacemaker placement. Causes that may increase this threshold include metabolic derangements (ie, electrolyte derangements[14,17,18]), antiarrhythmic drugs,[19–21] primary cardiomyopathies, myocardial infarction, or fibrosis at the electrode–myocardial interface. Modern electrodes are designed to minimize scar tissue generation that can cause higher thresholds during lead maturation or with exit blocks.

Failure to Pace (Output Failure)

Failure to pace describes when a pacer spike is expected but not generated. Depending on the programming of the pacemaker (asynchronous vs demand pacing), pacemakers may be continuously pacing or only pacing as needed. For example, in a demand pacemaker setting, it is normal and appropriate for there to be absence of pacemaker stimuli and pacemaker-generated depolarization so long as the patient's intrinsic conduction system is maintaining ventricular depolarization at or above the pacemaker's programmed base rate. If there are pause intervals longer than expected for a set base rate without a pacemaker stimulus, this is termed failure to pace. If these pauses are occurring but a pacemaker stimulus is seen without ventricular depolarization, this is a failure to capture. The difference between the 2 is illustrated in **Fig. 4**, which shows a paced QRS complexes followed by a pacer spike without subsequent myocardial depolarization (ie, failure to capture) followed by the absence of a paced stimulus when expected (ie, failure to pace).

A failure to pace can be a life-threatening problem, especially if there is severe conduction disease or if the individual is pacemaker dependent. The 2 most common reasons pacemakers fail to pace are due to oversensing (as above) or an open circuit

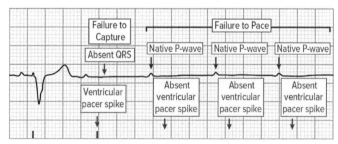

Fig. 4. This rhythm strip shows a paced QRS complex followed by failure to capture then failure to pace (ECG image courtesy of Jeremy G. Berberian, MD).

between the generator and the myocardium (eg, lead fracture or insulation defect, inadequate lead fixation).[15,16]

PACEMAKER-ASSOCIATED DYSRHYTHMIAS

Pacemaker mediated tachycardia (PMT), also called endless-loop tachycardia, is a reentry tachycardia that is very similar to antidromic AVRT, except that the pacemaker replaces the accessory pathway. It occurs with dual-chamber pacemakers that have atrial sensing. The typical trigger is a premature ventricular contraction that causes a retrograde P-wave that is sensed by the atrial lead, which then triggers ventricular depolarization, leading to another retrograde P-wave, and so forth. The antegrade impulse is via the pacemaker with retrograde conduction through the AV node. Dual-chamber pacemakers are programmed such that the atrial lead has a refractory period to prevent it from being retriggered by the ventricular depolarization or retrograde P-waves.[22] This is called the postventricular atrial refractory period, and PMT can occur if it is too brief. Treatment with either a magnet or nodal blocking agent will terminate the dysrhythmia.[4,23]

Runaway pacemaker is an excessive increase in pacing rate leading to potentially lethal ventricular rhythms and occurs in older generation pacemakers. This phenomenon is extremely rare and unlikely to persist given advancements in pacemaker technology and set upper limits in programming. If ever encountered, it is usually due to a component failure (eg, low battery) and is a medical emergency. Magnet application will typically cause the pacemaker to pace at a default rate, and emergent cardiac consultation is required for interrogation and attempted reprograming. As a last resort, surgical intervention to disconnect the leads could be considered.[24]

OTHER PEARLS AND PITFALLS

Pacemaker syndrome is a hemodynamic effect generated by a normal functioning pacemaker system programmed with single-chamber VVI pacing (rarely with DDD) and may occur in up to 25% of patients.[25] The AV dysynchrony results in loss of the atrial kick, which manifests as inadequate cardiac output and poor functional status. The syndrome represents a clinical spectrum and may present with a gamut of signs and symptoms of variable severity. Patients typically complain of fatigue, weakness, dyspnea, lightheadedness or dizziness, neck or throat discomfort, and atypical chest discomfort. Objective examination may reveal evidence of AV dissociation and heart failure such as cannon A waves and elevated jugular venous pressure (JVP), hypotension, rales, peripheral edema, and valvular insufficiency murmurs.[4,25,26] Note, this is not a failure of the pacemaker but an intolerance of the pacing mode. Patients' inability to tolerate VVI pacing may require upgrade to dual-chamber devices.[15,25]

Hysteresis is a programmable parameter within most pacemakers that often can be misinterpreted as failure to pace. The hysteresis parameter is programmed such that the interval between a native beat and the first paced escape beat is longer than the programmed base rate of the pacemaker. This allows patients with an intermittent pacing requirement to use their native rhythm instead of pacing unless they reach a predetermined critical threshold.[27] It is not a failure of the pulse generator or leads of the pacemaker. For example, a pacemaker with hysteresis may have a base rate of 80 bpm but will allow the rate to drop as low as 60 bpm before initiating pacing at the base rate of 80 bpm. This is usually identified by native heart rates lower than their base pacemaker rates or pauses established only after native cardiac depolarizations. This feature can be activated or deactivated by the cardiologist.

Fusion and pseudo-fusion complexes are ECG findings of competitive pacemaking between the intrinsic cardiac conduction system and the pacemaker. The fusion beat will have a mixed appearance between intrinsic conduction and pacemaker morphology because the pacemaker was able to depolarize the peri-electrode myocardium. If the pacemaker was not able to depolarize the myocardium, a pseudo-fusion beat will be seen that resembles the intrinsic conduction system.[5] These are normal occurrences and do not demonstrate pacemaker malfunction or failure.

ADVANCE CARDIAC LIFE SUPPORT WITH PACEMAKERS

Individuals with pacemakers may present critically ill with cardiac instability with or without pacemaker failure. Although external cardioversion and defibrillation are known to potentially cause malfunction with generators, leads, sensors, and electrodes,[28] it may also be a life-saving intervention. Special considerations should be considered when performing external electrical cardioversion or defibrillation.[29] First, consider if the procedure is necessary and emergent. If neither of these is applicable, discussion with the cardiologist before performing these actions is appropriate. Patients with a combined pacemaker and implantable cardioverter-defibrillator could receive cardioversion or defibrillation using the device instead of external shock if the cardiologist is available to coordinate care. If performing external electrical cardioversion or defibrillation, the following precautions have demonstrated safety and effectiveness in patients with pacemakers.[29] External pads or electrodes should be placed 8 to 12 cm from the pulse generator in the anterior–posterior configuration.[30] During cardioversion, the lowest energy indicated for the dysrhythmia should be used first to minimize the risk of damaging the device and internal electrode. After cardioversion or defibrillation is completed, device interrogation and evaluation by a cardiologist is required to ensure proper integrity and function. Return of pacing with capture may not occur immediately following defibrillation due to ischemia and increased pacing threshold.[4] If capture does not return spontaneously, transcutaneous pacing can be attempted until the device can be interrogated and reprogrammed by cardiology.

REPROGRAMMING IN CRITICALLY ILL

Devices may require reprogramming in critically ill patients for which the pacemaker may be contributing to the patient's condition. For example, patients experiencing or at risk for torsades de pointes may warrant emergent intervention by cardiology to reprogram the device to a base rate closer to 100 bpm to reduce the risk of R-on-T phenomena. Additionally, patients without rate responsiveness may not have optimal heart rates to meet physiologic demands in the setting of shock and may benefit from an increased heart rate to augment cardiac output.[31] Critically ill patients may also demonstrate inappropriate ventricular response to atrial dysrhythmias, and this can be resolved by reprogramming the device to single-chamber mode. Close communication and coordination with cardiology is recommended for optimizing hemodynamics in critically ill patients.

CASE CHALLENGE DISCUSSION

This ECG shows an atrial-sensed, ventricular-paced rhythm with an average ventricular rate of 36 bpm and frequent failure to capture, left axis deviation, and prolonged QRS complex duration with an LBBB-like morphology. Note that the QRS complex in lead V6 is negatively oriented, which is normal for single ventricle pacing. The

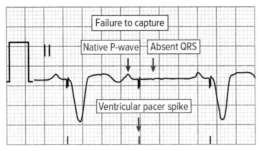

Fig. 5. Failure to capture. (ECG image courtesy of Jeremy G. Berberian, MD)

P-QRS-T complexes associated with the 1st, 3rd, 5th, 7th, 10th, and 12th pacer spikes show a normal atrial-sensed ventricular-paced rhythm-there is a native P-wave that is sensed by the pacemaker, which then triggers a paced ventricular beat. The 2nd, 4th, 6th, 8th, 9th, 11th, and 13th pacer spikes show no subsequent ventricular depolarization, which is consistent with failure to capture (**Fig. 5**). In this case, the underlying cause of the failure to capture was an increased capture threshold due to hyperkalemia.

SUMMARY

Modern pacemaker technology and design have optimized function and eliminated many issues encountered in the past but dysfunction and failure still occur. These malfunctions can occur at any site within the system from the pulse generator and leads to the electrode–myocardium interface. Pacemaker failures may be related to abnormal sensing, capture, and/or pacing. Malfunctions can have severe hemodynamic consequences so rapid identification of the specific dysfunction utilizing history, ECG, magnet application, chest radiograph, and cardiology consultation is critical in determining the appropriate interventions to stabilize the patient.

CLINICS CARE POINTS

- Pacemaker malfunction may result from any component of the device or the patient's intrinsic cardiac system.
- Electrocardiogram is essential in the emergency department evaluation of pacemaker function while metabolic panel, chest radiography, and cardiology consultation are important adjunctive steps.
- Magnets are diagnostic and therapeutic interventions that will temporarily cause the pacemaker to switch to asynchronous pacing.
- External pacing, cardioversion, and defibrillation are safe with permanent pacemakers when using anterior–posterior pad placement at least 8 to 12 cm from generator and use of the lowest energy required.
- Fusion beats, pseudofusion beats, and hysteresis are normal features that may be misidentified as pacemaker malfunctions.
- Pacemaker syndrome presents with variable complaints and should be suspected in someone with a single chamber, ventricularly paced device who has evidence of inadequate cardiac output and poor functional status.

DISCLOSURE

No relationships to disclose.

REFERENCES

1. Reddy VY, Exner DV, Cantillon DJ, et al. Percutaneous implantation of an entirely intracardiac leadless pacemaker. N Engl J Med 2015;373(12):1125–35.
2. Lau C-P, Chen K, Lee KL-F, et al. Implantation and clinical performance of an entirely leadless cardiac pacemaker. Int J Heart Rhythm 2016;1:50–4.
3. Maisel WH, Moynahan M, Zuckerman BD, et al. Pacemaker and ICD generator malfunctions: analysis of Food and Drug Administration annual reports. JAMA 2006;295(16):1901–6.
4. Squire B, Niemann J. Implantable Cardiac Devices. In: Walls RM, Hockberger RS, Gausche-Hill M, editors. Rosen's emergency medicine: concepts and clinical practice, 1, 9th Edition. Philadelphia, PA: Elsevier; 2018. p. 959–70.
5. Bagliani G, Sacchi S, Padeletti L. How tO INTERPRET PACEMAKER ELECTRO-CARDiograms. In: Al-Ahmad A, Natale A, Wang PJ, et al, editors. How-to manual for pacemaker and ICD devices: procedures and programming. Hoboken, NJ: John Wiley & Sons, Inc.; 2018. p. 159–72.
6. Bernstein AD, Daubert JC, Fletcher RD, et al. The revised NASPE/BPEG generic code for antibradycardia, adaptive-rate, and multisite pacing. North American Society of Pacing and Electrophysiology/British Pacing and Electrophysiology Group. Pacing Clin Electrophysiol 2002;25(2):260–4.
7. Kusumoto FM, Schoenfeld MH, Barrett C, et al. 2018 ACC/AHA/HRS Guideline on the Evaluation and Management of Patients With Bradycardia and Cardiac Conduction Delay: A Report of the American College of Cardiology/American Heart Association Task Force on Clinical Practice Guidelines and the Heart Rhythm Society. Circulation 2019;140(8):e382–482.
8. Lamas GA, Orav EJ, Stambler BS, et al. Quality of life and clinical outcomes in elderly patients treated with ventricular pacing as compared with dual-chamber pacing. Pacemaker Selection in the Elderly Investigators. N Engl J Med 1998; 338(16):1097–104.
9. Healey JS, Toff WD, Lamas GA, et al. Cardiovascular outcomes with atrial-based pacing compared with ventricular pacing: meta-analysis of randomized trials, using individual patient data. Circulation 2006;114(1):11–7.
10. Sweeney MO, Prinzen FW. A new paradigm for physiologic ventricular pacing. J Am Coll Cardiol 2006;47(2):282–8.
11. Curtis AB, Worley SJ, Adamson PB, et al. Biventricular pacing for atrioventricular block and systolic dysfunction. N Engl J Med 2013;368(17):1585–93.
12. Curtis AB, Worley SJ, Chung ES, et al. Improvement in clinical outcomes with biventricular versus right ventricular pacing: the BLOCK HF study. J Am Coll Cardiol 2016;67(18):2148–57.
13. Israel CW. Analysis of mode switching algorithms in dual chamber pacemakers. Pacing Clin Electrophysiol 2002;25(3):380–93.
14. Schiraldi F, Guiotto G, Paladino F. Hyperkalemia induced failure of pacemaker capture and sensing. Resuscitation 2008;79(1):161–4.
15. Murphy JG. Pacemakers; cardiac resynchronization therapy. In: Mayo clinic cardiology concise textbook. 4th edition. Oxford: Mayo Clinic Scientific Press; 2013. p. 324–38.

16. Cardall TY, Brady WJ, Chan TC, et al. Permanent cardiac pacemakers: issues relevant to the emergency physician, part II. J Emerg Med 1999;17(4):697–709.
17. Ortega-Carnicer J, Benezet J, Benezet-Mazuecos J. Hyperkalaemia causing loss of atrial capture and extremely wide QRS complex during DDD pacing. Resuscitation 2004;62(1):119–20.
18. Kahloon MU, Aslam AK, Aslam AF, et al. Hyperkalemia induced failure of atrial and ventricular pacemaker capture. Int J Cardiol 2005;105(2):224–6.
19. Van Herendael H, Pinter A, Ahmad K, et al. Role of antiarrhythmic drugs in patients with implantable cardioverter defibrillators. Europace 2010;12(5):618–25.
20. Hook BG, Perlman RL, Callans DJ, et al. Acute and chronic cycle length dependent increase in ventricular pacing threshold. Pacing Clin Electrophysiol 1992; 15(10 Pt 1):1437–44.
21. Rajawat YS, Patel VV, Gerstenfeld EP, et al. Advantages and pitfalls of combining device-based and pharmacologic therapies for the treatment of ventricular arrhythmias: observations from a tertiary referral center. Pacing Clin Electrophysiol 2004;27(12):1670–81.
22. Alasti M, Machado C, Rangasamy K, et al. Pacemaker-mediated arrhythmias. J Arrhythm 2018;34(5):485–92.
23. Barold SS. Repetitive reentrant and non-reentrant ventriculoatrial synchrony in dual chamber pacing. Clin Cardiol 1991;14(9):754–63.
24. Griffin J, Smithline H, Cook J. Runaway pacemaker: a case report and review. J Emerg Med 2000;19(2):177–81.
25. Glikson M, Nielsen JC, Kronborg MB, et al. 2021 ESC Guidelines on cardiac pacing and cardiac resynchronization therapy. Eur Heart J 2021;42(35):3427–520.
26. Ausubel K, Furman S. The pacemaker syndrome. Ann Intern Med 1985;103(3): 420–9.
27. García-Izquierdo E, Vilches S, Castro V. Is This Pacemaker Functioning Abnormally? Circulation 2017;135(7):711–3.
28. Waller C, Callies F, Langenfeld H. Adverse effects of direct current cardioversion on cardiac pacemakers and electrodes Is external cardioversion contraindicated in patients with permanent pacing systems? Europace 2004;6(2):165–8.
29. Manegold JC, Israel CW, Ehrlich JR, et al. External cardioversion of atrial fibrillation in patients with implanted pacemaker or cardioverter-defibrillator systems: a randomized comparison of monophasic and biphasic shock energy application. Eur Heart J 2007;28(14):1731–8.
30. Levine PA, Barold SS, Fletcher RD, et al. Adverse acute and chronic effects of electrical defibrillation and cardioversion on implanted unipolar cardiac pacing systems. J Am Coll Cardiol 1983;1(6):1413–22.
31. McPherson CA, Manthous C. Permanent pacemakers and implantable defibrillators: considerations for intensivists. Am J Respir Crit Care Med 2004;170(9): 933–40.

Management of Acute Coronary Syndrome

Joel Atwood, MD

KEYWORDS

- Acute coronary syndrome • Myocardial infarction
- ST segment elevation myocardial infarction
- Non-ST segment elevation myocardial infarction • Unstable angina

KEY POINTS

- The underlying cause of cardiac ischemia directs management.
- Early identification and revascularization of patients with ST-Segment elevation myocardial infarction improve outcomes.
- All patients with suspected or confirmed acute coronary syndrome (ACS) should immediately receive aspirin.
- Emergency providers should identify and treat early complications of ACS.

DEFINITIONS

An acute coronary syndrome (ACS) is caused by coronary plaque rupture/erosion and thrombus formation leading to obstruction of blood flow and distal myocardial ischemia.[1,2] The degree of coronary artery obstruction and cardiac ischemia highlight the pathophysiological differences between the clinical entities of ST-Segment elevation myocardial infarction (STEMI), Non-ST-Segment elevation myocardial infarction (NSTEMI), and unstable angina (UA). In STEMI, the coronary artery is completely or nearly occluded resulting in evidence of transmural ischemia on electrocardiogram (ECG) (ST-segment elevation), symptoms of angina, and myocardial cell death on troponin assays. In NSTEMI, the coronary artery is at least partially occluded resulting in subendocardial ischemia, symptoms of angina, and myocardial cell death; however, there are no ST-segment elevations on ECG. In UA, the coronary artery thrombus results in symptoms or ECG changes typical of myocardial ischemia; however, there is no measurable myocardial cell death (**Fig. 1**).

Although ACS is the primary concern for most providers when encountering a patient with compatible symptoms, alternative pathologies leading to myocardial injury are common. Causes are numerous and result in any circumstance where myocardial

Department of Emergency Medicine, 1300 South George Street, York, PA 17402, USA
E-mail address: jatwood@wellspan.org

Emerg Med Clin N Am 40 (2022) 693–706
https://doi.org/10.1016/j.emc.2022.06.008
0733-8627/22/© 2022 Elsevier Inc. All rights reserved.

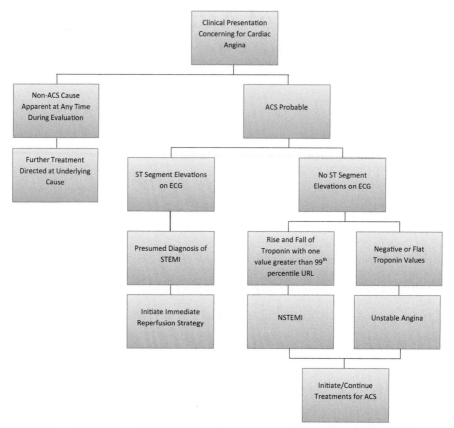

Fig. 1. Conceptualization of ACS. ACS, acute coronary syndrome; ECG, electrocardiogram; NSTEMI, non-ST segment myocardial infarction; STEMI, ST-segment elevation myocardial infarction; URL, upper reference limit.

oxygen demands exceed supply. Common examples include coronary vasospasm, sepsis, and anemia (**Fig. 2**). After a provider identifies evidence of myocardial ischemia by history, ECG, or laboratories, a rapid evaluation to determine the underlying cause is imperative. Treatment of non-ACS causes of myocardial ischemia is directed at correcting the underlying abnormality that created the oxygen imbalance. Typical ACS strategies are unlikely to be helpful and more likely to result in iatrogenic harm in these circumstances. In this article, we focus on the treatment of acute myocardial ischemia caused by ACS.

INITIAL APPROACH TO ACUTE CORONARY SYNDROME MANAGEMENT

After the emergency clinician diagnoses ACS, simultaneous efforts to improve and prevent worsening of oxygen mismatch are initiated. The time course of strategies is dictated by the type of ACS encountered (STEMI vs. NSTEMI vs. UA) as well as patient-specific factors, including comorbidities, medications, bleeding risk, and duration of symptoms. In addition to supportive care, the approach to treatment is directed at optimizing myocardial ischemia through three different mechanisms:

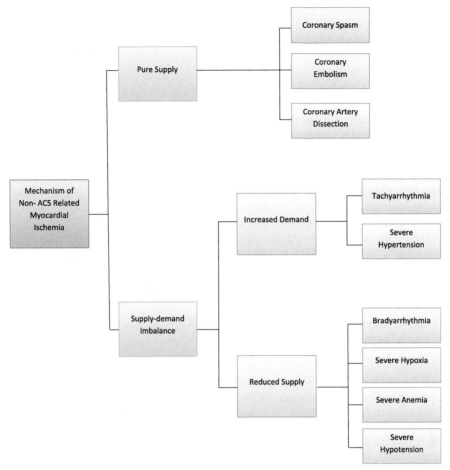

Fig. 2. Pathophysiology of type 2 myocardial infarction. (This article was published in Journal of the American College of Cardiology, 70(13), Januzzi JL, Sandoval Y, The Many Faces of Type 2 Myocardial Infarction, 1569–1572, Copyright Elsevier 2017.)

- Improving myocardial oxygen imbalance
- Decreasing coronary artery thrombus propagation
- Coronary artery reperfusion through revascularization

OPTIMIZING OXYGEN DELIVERY

It has been previously taught that all patients suffering from ACS should be started on supplemental oxygen to improve oxygen delivery to the ischemic myocardium. However, standard use of oxygen is potentially detrimental because hyperoxia can cause coronary vasoconstriction and increased oxidative stress. Randomized trials have not shown the benefits of routine oxygen supplementation and potential harm.[3] Currently, oxygen is only recommended when levels drop below 90% or in cases of respiratory distress.[4]

Anemia is common in patients with ACS with up to 10% of patients requiring a blood transfusion during hospitalization.[5] Although transfusion will increase oxygen carry capacity and myocardial oxygen supply, side effects include increased thrombogenesis and volume overload. For these reasons, there is continued debate regarding the appropriate transfusion threshold. Routine transfusion beginning at a hemoglobin level of 8 g/dL is reasonable.[6]

DECREASING MYOCARDIAL DEMAND

Ischemic pain and anxiety should be treated to alleviate symptoms as well as decrease myocardial oxygen demand generated from sympathetic nervous system activation and increased work of breathing. Nitroglycerin improves coronary perfusion and decreases cardiac preload and afterload, relieving ischemic discomfort. Nitroglycerin should be avoided in patients with concerns for right ventricular ischemia, ongoing hypotension, recent phosphodiesterase use, or known aortic stenosis. In suitable patients who have improved with sublingual nitroglycerin treatment, a low dose infusion titrated to pain or systolic blood pressure is indicated.

Liberal use of morphine for patients with ischemic discomfort was previously encouraged; however, studies suggest morphine and other opiates, such as fentanyl impact early $P2Y_{12}$ antiplatelet agent metabolism which has been associated with early treatment failures.[7,8] For this reason, morphine and other opiates should be used judiciously in refractory pain. Treatment with low-dose benzodiazepines is reasonable in appropriate patients.[4]

Hypertension is common in patients presenting with ACS and results in increased myocardial oxygen demand. Early and aggressive use of IV beta-blockers to reduce hypertension, cardiac contractility, and heart rate results in lower rates of recurrent myocardial infarction and ventricular fibrillation (VF) but higher rates of early cardiogenic shock.[9] Risk factors for beta-blocker-induced cardiogenic shock include advanced age (>70), tachycardia, systolic blood pressures less than 120, or evidence of heart failure on presentation. IV beta-blockers are commonly avoided because of concerns of iatrogenic harm; however, it is appropriate to treat select ACS patients with refractory pain and hypertension with IV metoprolol.[10]

SUPPORTIVE CARE

All patients with ACS should have reliable IV access and continuous telemetry and pulse oximetry monitoring to detect abnormalities so that providers can intervene at the first sign of decompensation. Electrolyte derangements are associated with arrhythmias, thus it is recommended to routinely administer potassium and magnesium to goal levels of 4.0 mEq/L and 2.0 mEq/L, respectively.

ST SEGMENT ELEVATION MYOCARDIAL INFARCTION
Initial Identification

Early identification and evaluation for STEMI are of pivotal importance as rapid treatment improves outcomes.[11] An ECG should be obtained within 10 minutes of first medical contact.[10] A presumptive diagnosis of STEMI requires a history consistent with cardiac angina and a compatible ECG (**Box 1**). The diagnosis of STEMI is finalized when the left heart catheterization reveals evidence of an acutely occluded artery. In patients treated with a noninvasive revascularization approach, the diagnosis is confirmed by new ischemic Q waves, evidence of ischemia on imaging, or a typical rise and fall of troponin levels.[12]

Box 1
Definition of ST segment elevation on ECG

New ST-segment elevation at the J-point in two contiguous leads

ST-segment elevation is defined as $\geq$1.0 mm in all leads other than V_2–V_3, V_3R–V_4R, and V_7–V_9

ST-segment elevation definitions in leads V_2-V_3 vary by patient age/sex
    $\geq$2.5 mm in men less than 40 years of age
    $\geq$2 mm in men $\geq$ 40 years of age
    $\geq$1.5 mm in women regardless of age

ST-Segment elevation definitions in leads V_3R and V_4R vary by patient age/sex
    $\geq$0.5 mm in men $\geq$ 30 years of age and all women
    $\geq$1.0 mm in men less than 30 years of age

ST-Segment elevation is defined as $\geq$ 0.5 mm in leads V_7–V_9

Abbreviation: ECG, electrocardiogram.

Data from Thygesen K, Alpert JS, Jaffe AS, et al. Fourth Universal Definition of Myocardial Infarction (2018). J Am Coll Cardiol. 2018;72(18):2231-2264. https://doi.org/10.1016/j.jacc. 2018.08.1038 and Wagner GS, MacFarlane P, Wellens H, et al. AHA/ACCF/HRS recommendations for the standardization and interpretation of the electrocardiogram: Part VI: Acute ischemia/ infarction: A scientific statement from the American Heart Association Electrocardiography and Arrhythmias Committee, Council on Clinical Cardiology; The American College of Cardiology Foundation; And the Heart Rhythm Society. Circulation. 2009;119(10):262-270. https://doi. org/10.1161/CIRCULATIONAHA.108.191098.

Approach to Revascularization

Once a patient with STEMI is identified, the efforts to restore coronary artery perfusion via percutaneous coronary intervention (PCI) or fibrinolytic therapy should be initiated immediately. Primary PCI is the proven superior treatment in patients with STEMI because it is associated with lower rates of recurrent myocardial infarction, stroke, and death.[13] PCI is a highly technical, resource-intensive procedure, which is not available in all settings. When PCI cannot be accomplished within 120 minutes of first medical contact, fibrinolytic therapy should be administered in appropriate patients.[10]

Preparing Patient for Percutaneous Coronary Intervention

The primary responsibility of the emergency provider is to ensure the patient is stable to tolerate PCI and administration of appropriate medications. The rapid evaluation includes an assessment of the patient's airway, respiratory status (including the ability to comfortably lay supine), hemodynamics, and ability to cooperate and follow commands. There should be a low threshold to initiate aggressive supportive care measures, such as noninvasive positive pressure ventilation or endotracheal intubation to decrease the risk of untimely decompensation during left heart catheterization.

Early Medications for Patients Undergoing Percutaneous Coronary Intervention

Antithrombotic medications are administered to prevent thrombus propagation as well as iatrogenic complications during PCI. All patients presenting with suspected STEMI should receive aspirin. This low-risk intervention saves one life for every 42 patients treated.[14] Ideally, enteric-coated aspirin is avoided and the tablet should be chewed or crushed rather than swallowed. Rectal aspirin should be administered to patients who are unable to take it orally.

An additional antiplatelet $P2Y_{12}$ inhibitor is recommended for all patients treated for STEMI with PCI. These medications, which include clopidogrel, ticagrelor, prasugrel, and cangrelor, are proven to further decrease the risk of thrombotic complications. In most cases of STEMI, ticagrelor or prasugrel is recommended with head-to-head trials showing a slight advantage of prasugrel in carefully selected patients.[15] $P2Y_{12}$ inhibitor use must be balanced with an individual patient bleeding risk. Patients at higher risk of hemorrhage should receive clopidogrel.[16] Whereas there are theoretic benefits to early $P2Y_{12}$ inhibitor use and many protocols recommend these agents be given routinely in the emergency department, administration before angiogram has never been shown to be superior to the administration at the time of PCI. Accordingly, it is not unreasonable to defer the drug selection and administration by the interventional cardiologist.[10] In cases where there is high suspicion for proximal left anterior descending artery occlusion or left main coronary artery occlusion on ECG, the decision to start a second antiplatelet agent should be made at the time of angiogram, as these patients are at high risk for requiring coronary artery bypass grafting (CABG) procedures and PGY_{12} use before CABG significantly increases the risk of hemorrhagic complications.

Anticoagulation is recommended in all patients with STEMI undergoing a PCI revascularization strategy. The two most commonly used agents are unfractionated heparin and bivalirudin. Fondaparinux is associated with increased periprocedural thrombotic complications and is not recommended.[17] Low molecular weight heparin has not been studied extensively in the modern era of STEMI PCI management. Results from randomized trials between unfractionated heparin and bivalirudin reveal subtle differences between bleeding risk and thrombotic complications that are influenced by the site of arterial puncture, patient risk of bleeding, and other antithrombotic agent selection.[16] Both agents are reasonable choices and clinicians should follow institutional protocols or cardiology recommendations.

GP IIb/IIIa receptor antagonists work to inhibit the glycoprotein activation site and thus prevent platelet activation. Before the routine use of $P2Y_{12}$ inhibitors, there was evidence that routine early use of these agents decreased mortality.[18] However, in the $P2Y_{12}$ inhibitor era, additional GP IIb/IIIa receptor antagonists have not shown to have a meaningful difference with the two most widely available agents (tirofiban and eptifibatide) and are not routinely recommended before angiography.[10]

Fibrinolytic Reperfusion Strategy

In nonprimary PCI centers, even with close transport times, up to one-third of patients are unable to achieve guideline-directed PCI within 120 minutes of first medical contact.[19] Unexpected events within a primary center also can result in an inability to perform PCI, thus all emergency providers should be prepared to pursue a fibrinolytic strategy. Fibrin-specific agents (alteplase, reteplase, and tenecteplase) are the preferred agents for treating STEMI.[20] Teneceteplase may have a lower bleeding risk when compared with other agents.[21] The less expensive, but less efficacious, nonfibrin-specific agent streptokinase is still used in many parts of the world.

The risk profile of fibrinolytic therapy differs from PCI; so, a rapid evaluation should be performed that weighs the benefits of fibrinolysis against the potential risks of hemorrhage. Patients who present immediately after symptom onset, are less than 65 year old, have a low bleeding risk profile, and are hemodynamically stable will benefit the most. Reperfusion through fibrinolytic therapy should be performed within 30 minutes of arrival.[10] Given an estimated risk of intracranial bleeding of 1% with systemic fibrinolytic therapy, a careful evaluation for contraindications should be performed rapidly[22](**Box 2**). The patient should understand the risks and benefits of therapy and agree to treatment.

Box 2
Contraindications and precautions to fibrinolytic therapy

Contraindications
  Active internal bleeding
  Recent (within 3 months) intracranial or intraspinal surgery or serious head trauma
  Intracranial conditions that may increase the risk of bleeding (neoplasm, AV malformation,
  aneurysm, prior intracranial hemorrhage)
  Bleeding diathesis
  Current severe uncontrolled hypertension (SBP >180 and/or DBP >110)

Warning and Precautions
  Recent major surgery or procedure
  Known prior cerebrovascular disease
  Recent gastrointestinal or genitourinary bleeding
  Significant hepatic dysfunction or renal dysfunction
  Pregnancy
  Recent trauma
  Major surgery or puncture of noncompressible vessels

Abbreviations: AV, arteriovnenous; DBP, diastolic blood pressure; SBP, systolic blood pressure.

Data from Alteplase. Package insert. Genentech Pharmaceuticals. 2018.

Adjunctive Medications During Fibrinolysis

All patients should receive aspirin. Clopidogrel is the only $P2Y_{12}$ inhibitor studied in patients receiving fibrinolytic therapy and is recommended as it improves outcomes. Alternative $P2Y_{12}$ inhibitors and GIIb/IIIa receptor antagonists are not recommended given their documented increased risk of hemorrhage in other STEMI populations.[20] Anticoagulation with unfractionated or low molecular weight heparin is generally recommended.[23]

Post-Fibrinolytic Care

In the immediate post-fibrinolysis period successful treatment is indicated by decreased chest pain, stable hemodynamics, and improvement in ST elevations at 60 to 90 minutes.[23] Accelerated idioventricular reperfusion arrhythmias are common and do not cause clinical instability or require treatment. After fibrinolytic therapy is initiated, immediate transfer to a PCI center is recommended as treatment failures should receive urgent rescue PCI and most patients with treatment success also benefit from PCI within 24 hours.[24,25]

Delayed Presentation

Delayed presentation of STEMI is common. All patients with STEMI presenting in shock should undergo immediate revascularization regardless of the duration of symptoms.[10] Outside of this subset of patients there is no strong consensus on the utility of emergency revascularization. Early trials of revascularization with fibrinolysis in patients presenting greater than 12 hours after symptom onset failed to show a benefit. Emergency PCI in patients presenting within 12 to 48 hours of symptom onset has demonstrated prognostic benefits but there are no robust well-powered randomized trials to definitively guide emergency treatment.[26] Currently, guidelines recommend emergency PCI in patients presenting within 12 to 24 hours of pain that have clinical signs of ongoing ischemia. Carefully selected STEMI patients with 12 to 24 hours of symptoms and large areas of myocardium at risk may also be reasonable candidates for fibrinolytic therapy.[10] Management of asymptomatic patients or presentations of STEMI with less than 3 days of symptoms is even less well defined because a completed myocardial infarction would not benefit from emergency reperfusion. Routine revascularization of STEMI patients with greater than 3 days of symptoms is not beneficial.[27] After discussion with a cardiologist, select patients with delayed presentations of STEMI may be hospitalized for medical management, further provocative testing, or delayed PCI rather than emergently revascularized.

NON-ST-SEGMENT ELEVATION MYOCARDIAL INFARCTION AND UNSTABLE ANGINA

Overall acute management of patients presenting with NSTEMI and UA differs from STEMI in that emergency revascularization is rarely required. Initial antithrombotic approaches initiated in the ED also vary.

Antiplatelet and Antithrombotic Agents

All patients with NSTEMI and UA should be given aspirin as soon as possible. In contrast to patients with STEMI, routine upfront use of $P2Y_{12}$ agents is discouraged in patients receiving invasive revascularization strategies because trials have shown an increased risk of hemorrhage without any benefit.[28] A second agent can be administered after coronary angiography clarifies the anatomy and before PCI.[4] In some settings, dual antiplatelet therapy at the time of diagnosis may be reasonable, such as when a noninvasive strategy or delayed invasive strategy for the treatment of ACS is pursued. Prasugrel or ticagrelor are preferred over clopidogrel.[4] Similarly, GPIIb/IIIa receptor antagonists are not recommended routinely at the time of diagnosis in the emergency department.

Anticoagulation with unfractionated heparin, low molecular weight heparin, bivalirudin, or fondaparinux therapy is routinely recommended for all patients diagnosed with NSTEMI. There is no one anticoagulant that has a clear advantage when compared with others in every common patient scenario and the selection of the appropriate agent is complex. Factors that influence agent decision include bleeding risk, interaction with other therapies, plans for invasive versus medical management, time to an angiogram, and procedural technique. Agent selection is generally guided by institutional protocols or cardiology consultation.

Indications for Emergency Revascularization

Trials have failed to show an immediate benefit of emergency revascularization with PCI or fibrinolytic therapy in patients with NSTEMI. When an invasive revascularization strategy is pursued it is reasonable to perform PCI within 24 to 72 hours of presentation depending on patient factors.[29] However, very high-risk NSTEMI patients were excluded from previous trials and have a poor prognosis. They should be treated analogously to STEMI patients with emergency PCI[4] (**Box 3**).

MANAGEMENT OF ACUTE COMPLICATION OF ACUTE CORONARY SYNDROME
Electrical Complications

Ventricular arrhythmia in ACS carries a greater mortality risk and occurs in up to 5% of patients.[30] Immediate management includes cardioversion/defibrillation in unstable patients. Emergency revascularization, preferably via PCI is indicated to correct the underlying ischemia triggering the arrhythmia. Antiarrhythmic use in early ACS is largely driven by expert consensus. Beta-blockers should be initiated in otherwise stable patients to decrease sympathetic tone and decrease reoccurrence. Potassium and magnesium should be repleted to goal levels of 4.0 to 5.0 mEq/L and 2.0 mEq/L.[31]

Box 3
Indications for emergency PCI in NSTEMI
Hemodynamic instability/cardiogenic shock
Recurrent/refractory chest pain despite treatment
Life-threatening arrhythmia
Mechanical complications of MI
Acute heart failure clearly caused by ACS
ST-Segment depression greater than 1 mm in six leads plus ST-segment elevation in AVr and/or V1 clearly caused by ACS
Abbreviations: ACS, acute coronary syndrome; MI, myocardial infarction.
Data from Collet JP, Thiele H, Barbato E, et al. 2020 ESC Guidelines for the management of acute coronary syndromes in patients presenting without persistent ST-segment elevation. Eur Heart J. 2021;42(14):1289-1367. https://doi.org/10.1093/eurheartj/ehaa575.

Recurrent ventricular tachycardia/VF in ACS should be treated similarly to other patients with electrical storms, including the use of antiarrhythmic therapy (most commonly amiodarone).[31]

Bradycardia in early ACS is common and results from increased vagal tone or ischemia to the cardiac conduction system. In the absence of hemodynamic instability, no treatment is needed and most cases will resolve over time with treatment of ACS. When hemodynamically significant, initial medical treatment with atropine is indicated. Frequently high-grade heart blocks will not respond to atropine, and in these cases, transcutaneous or transvenous pacing is indicated while arranging emergency revascularization. Sympathomimetic agents to increase heart rate are sometimes necessary but generally avoided because they may exacerbate coronary malperfusion and increase cardiac oxygen demand.

Cardiogenic Shock and Acute Heart Failure

Acute heart failure and cardiogenic shock not caused by dysrhythmias in the immediate ACS period have a differential diagnosis that includes severe left ventricular heart dysfunction, acute mitral valve insufficiency, ventricular/septal wall rupture, and acute right heart failure. Rapid evaluation with bedside echocardiography is beneficial when the underlying diagnosis is not clear. An emergency cardiology consultation should be obtained because most patients will require emergency revascularization or cardiac surgery.

Left Ventricular Failure

A cardiogenic shock from left ventricular pump failure has a mortality rate of 50%.[32] Most patients with ACS that develop cardiogenic shock will have a STEMI but shock can occur in NSTEMI patients as well. Revascularization with PCI is recommended as soon as possible, even for patients with delayed presentations greater than 12 hours.[10] An initial attempt to improve hemodynamics with a 250 cc bolus of isotonic fluid is reasonable in patients without pulmonary edema or respiratory distress. Practitioners should rapidly escalate to vasopressor therapy if there is continued hemodynamic instability and evidence of malperfusion.

Vasopressor selection is variable and there is no high-quality data to recommend one agent over another. Norepinephrine is generally recommended as a first-line agent as dopamine has been associated with worse outcomes in cardiogenic shock.[33] It is prudent to use the lowest dose possible to achieve hemodynamic stability and minimize iatrogenic coronary vasoconstriction. In cases of continued malperfusion with stable blood pressures, a trial of dobutamine can be considered. Diuretics and afterload reducers are rarely used in the emergency department for ACS-induced cardiogenic shock and are generally considered in more stable patients when additional data clarify the hemodynamic state. Intra-aortic balloon pumps, left ventricular assist devices, and extracorporeal membrane oxygenation do not have a strong evidence base but are frequently used in refractory cases of a cardiogenic shock given the high mortality rate and limited treatment options.

Acute mitral valve insufficiency should be suspected in cardiogenic shock or acute pulmonary edema, particularly in the presence of a new systolic heart murmur. Rapid dilation of mitral annulus due to left ventricular dilation, ischemia to the valve leaflet, or papillary muscle/chordae tendineae rupture are the main causes and are readily identified on cardiac ultrasound. When there is evidence of papillary muscle/chordae tendineae rupture, emergency cardiac surgery consultation is recommended for repair. In other cases, emergency revascularization is indicated and potentially curative. Acute afterload reducing agents are recommended in hemodynamically stable patients awaiting definitive care.

Myocardial wall rupture is generally seen with delayed presentations of ACS because prolonged periods of ischemia result in large areas of infarcted myocardium. Depending on the location of the rupture, a pericardial effusion (left ventricular free wall) or left to right shunt (intraventricular septum) can result. These events are often rapidly fatal and emergency cardiac surgery consultation is recommended. If hemodynamics permits, a rapid decrease in afterload is recommended to maximize blood flow through the aorta in addition to supportive care.

Acute right-sided heart failure is suspected in ACS when the patient presents with hypotension, distended neck veins, and evidence of a right-sided infarct on ECG. Initial stabilization while arranging emergency revascularization includes a rapid infusion of intravenous fluids to support right ventricular preload.[10]

UNIQUE CIRCUMSTANCES IN ACUTE CORONARY SYNDROME MANAGEMENT
Geriatric Patients

ACS is more common in geriatric patients and their presentations can be subtle, leading to delays in diagnosis and treatment. It is well documented that geriatric patients are also at higher risk of short- and long-term outcomes from ACS and its treatment side effects, including hemorrhage, heart failure, and death.[34] Overall management of ACS in the elderly is similar to younger patients. A provider should have a heightened level of awareness of comorbidities, which may impact the selection and dosing of medications as well as the downstream therapeutic approach. Age is cited as one of the leading reasons a more conservative approach to care is pursued; however, age alone should not be the sole determination in this decision. Invasive strategies have been shown to improve outcomes for patients in their 80s and 90s.[35]

Cardiac Arrest

It is well established that patients with STEMI who are resuscitated from cardiac arrest should have emergency PCI once stabilized.[36] When there is no evidence of STEMI on ECG after cardiac arrest, the indications for emergency PCI are not clear. Many patients with cardiac arrest will have coronary artery disease; however, less than 25% of these patients actually have a new culprit lesion that explains their presentation.

Routine emergency PCI in the post-arrest period has not been shown to improve outcomes in randomized trials.[37] In practice, the available patient history (eg, preceding chest pain), known comorbidities, initial heart rhythm, evidence of ongoing ischemia, and early prognostication are all considered when deciding on an emergency PCI strategy.[38]

Cocaine

Cocaine use can lead to acute coronary ischemia through multiple mechanisms including coronary vasoconstriction and increased myocardial oxygen demand from sympathetic stimulation as well as inciting acute plaque rupture or spontaneous thrombogenesis.[39] Risk of ACS is highest in the immediate post-ingestion period.[40] Once a diagnosis of ACS is established management is similar to ACS in other situations with the following exceptions. Liberal use of nitroglycerin is encouraged to relieve coronary constriction and high doses of benzodiazepines should be administered if there is evidence of a sympathomimetic toxidrome (eg, agitation, tachycardia, hypertension). Although there is no robust evidence, most practitioners avoid beta-blockers due to concerns about triggering unopposed alpha stimulation leading to coronary vasoconstriction.

SUMMARY

Patients are diagnosed with ACS routinely on every shift. The range or presentation includes the subtle symptoms in the well-appearing patients to the overtly critically ill in the patient with ischemia-induced shock. Cornerstones of management include aggressive supportive care, early optimization of myocardial mismatch, prevention of thrombus propagation, and improving early perfusion with PCI or fibrinolytic agents in select patients.

CLINICS CARE POINTS

- All patients with chest pain should have an electrocardiogram (ECG) within 10 minutes to evaluate for ST-Segment elevation myocardial infarction (STEMI).

- All patients with suspected acute coronary syndrome (ACS) should receive aspirin as soon as possible.

- All patients with ongoing or recurrent chest pain concerning for ACS should have serial ECGs to evaluate for evolution of myocardial infarction and STEMI.

- Patients with STEMI should have revascularization (fibrinolytics vs. percutaneous coronary intervention) as soon as possible.

- Follow institutional guidelines regarding additional antiplatelet agents and anticoagulation because recommendations vary according to typical downstream management patterns.

- Avoid routine use of oxygen and morphine in patients with ACS.

DISCLOSURE

The author has nothing to disclose.

REFERENCES

1. Weiss AJ, Ph D, Wier LM, et al. STATISTICAL BRIEF # 174 in the United States, 2011. 2014;(May 2013):1-13.

2. Wong KE, Divya Parikh P, Miller KC, et al. Emergency department and urgent care medical malpractice claims 2001-15. West J Emerg Med 2021;22(2):333–8.

3. Stub D, Smith K, Bernard S, et al. Air versus oxygen in ST-segment-elevation myocardial infarction. Circulation 2015;131(24):2143–50.

4. Collet JP, Thiele H, Barbato E, et al. 2020 ESC Guidelines for the management of acute coronary syndromes in patients presenting without persistent ST-segment elevation. Eur Heart J 2021;42(14):1289–367.

5. Jollis JG, Harrington R a, Granger CB, et al. Relationship of Blood Transfusion. October. 2004;292(13):1555-1562. Available at: http://www.ncbi.nlm.nih.gov/pubmed/15467057. Accessed January 10, 2022.

6. Ducrocq G, Gonzalez-Juanatey JR, Puymirat E, et al. Effect of a Restrictive vs Liberal Blood Transfusion Strategy on Major Cardiovascular Events among Patients with Acute Myocardial Infarction and Anemia: The REALITY Randomized Clinical Trial. JAMA 2021;325(6):552–60.

7. Parodi G, Bellandi B, Xanthopoulou I, et al. Morphine is associated with a delayed activity of oral antiplatelet agents in patients with st-elevation acute myocardial infarction undergoing primary percutaneous coronary intervention. Circ Cardiovasc Interv 2015;8(1):1–6.

8. McEvoy JW, Ibrahim K, Kickler TS, et al. Effect of intravenous fentanyl on ticagrelor absorption and platelet inhibition among patients undergoing percutaneous coronary intervention: The PACIFY randomized clinical trial (platelet aggregation with ticagrelor inhibition and fentanyl). Circulation 2018;137(3):307–9.

9. Chen Z, Xie J. Early intravenous then oral metoprolol in 45 852 patients with acute myocardial infarction: Randomised placebo-controlled trial. Lancet 2005;366(9497):1622–32.

10. Anderson JL. 2013 ACCF/AHA guideline for the management of ST-elevation myocardial infarction: A report of the American College of Cardiology Foundation/American Heart Association Task Force on practice guidelines. Circulation 2013;127(4):362–425.

11. Park J, Choi KH, Lee JM, et al. Prognostic Implications of Door-to-Balloon Time and Onset-to-Door Time on Mortality in Patients With ST-Segment–Elevation Myocardial Infarction Treated With Primary Percutaneous Coronary Intervention. J Am Heart Assoc 2019;8(9). https://doi.org/10.1161/JAHA.119.012188.

12. Thygesen K, Alpert JS, Jaffe AS, et al. Fourth Universal Definition of Myocardial Infarction (2018). J Am Coll Cardiol 2018;72(18):2231–64.

13. Keeley EC, Boura JA, Grines CL. Primary angioplasty versus intravenous thrombolytic therapy for acute myocardial infarction: A quantitative review of 23 randomised trials. Lancet 2003;361(9351):13–20.

14. Trial C. Randomised Trial of Intravenous Streptokinase, Oral Aspirin, Both, or Neither Among 17 187 Cases of Suspected Acute Myocardial Infarction: Isis-2. Lancet 1988;332(8607):349–60.

15. Schüpke S, Neumann F-J, Menichelli M, et al. Ticagrelor or Prasugrel in Patients with Acute Coronary Syndromes. N Engl J Med 2019;381(16):1524–34.

16. National Institute for Health and Care Excellence. Acute Coronary Syndromes. 2020. Available at: https://www.nice.org.uk/guidance/ng185. Accessed January 10, 2022.

17. Yusuf S. Effects of fondaparinux on mortality and reinfarction in patients with acute ST-segment elevation myocardial infarction: The OASIS-6 randomized trial. J Am Med Assoc 2006;295(13):1519–30.

18. De Luca G, Suryapranata H, Stone GW, et al. Abciximab as adjunctive therapy to reperfusion in acute ST-segment elevation myocardial infarction: A meta-analysis of randomized trials. J Am Med Assoc 2005;293(14):1759–65.

19. Vora AN, Holmes DN, Rokos I, et al. Fibrinolysis use among patients requiring interhospital transfer for st-segment elevation myocardial infarction care a report from the us national cardiovascular data registry. JAMA Intern Med 2015; 175(2):207–15.

20. Jinatongthai P, Kongwatcharapong J, Foo CY, et al. Comparative efficacy and safety of reperfusion therapy with fibrinolytic agents in patients with ST-segment elevation myocardial infarction: a systematic review and network meta-analysis. Lancet 2017;390(10096):747–59.

21. Guillermin A, Yan DJ, Perrier A, et al. Safety and efficacy of tenecteplase versus alteplase in acute coronary syndrome: A systematic review and meta-Analysis of randomized trials. Arch Med Sci 2016;12(6):1181–7.

22. Brass LM, Lichtman JH, Wang Y, et al. Intracranial hemorrhage associated with thrombolytic therapy for elderly patients with acute myocardial infarction: Results from the cooperative cardiovascular project. Stroke 2000;31(8):1802–11.

23. Engel Gonzalez P, Omar W, Patel KV, et al. Fibrinolytic Strategy for ST-Segment-Elevation Myocardial Infarction: A Contemporary Review in Context of the COVID-19 Pandemic. Circ Cardiovasc Interv 2020;81–8. https://doi.org/10.1161/CIRCINTERVENTIONS.120.009622.

24. Cantor WJ, Fitchett D, Borgundvaag B, et al. Routine Early Angioplasty after Fibrinolysis for Acute Myocardial Infarction. N Engl J Med 2009;360(26):2705–18.

25. Gershlick AH, Stephens-Lloyd A, Hughes S, et al. Rescue Angioplasty after Failed Thrombolytic Therapy for Acute Myocardial Infarction. N Engl J Med 2005;353(26):2758–68.

26. Schömig A, Mehilli J, Antoniucci D, et al. Mechanical reperfusion in patients with acute myocardial infarction presenting more than 12 hours from symptom onset: A randomized controlled trial. J Am Med Assoc 2005;293(23):2865–72.

27. Hochman JS, Lamas GA, Buller CE, et al. Coronary Intervention for Persistent Occlusion after Myocardial Infarction. N Engl J Med 2006;355(23):2395–407.

28. Montalescot G, Bolognese L, Dudek D, et al. Pretreatment with Prasugrel in Non–ST-Segment Elevation Acute Coronary Syndromes. N Engl J Med 2013;369(11):999–1010.

29. Collet C, Serruys PW. Early invasive strategy should be performed within 72 hours in high-risk patients with non-ST-elevation myocardial infarction. Evid Based Med 2017;22(6):227.

30. Mehta RH, Starr AZ, Lopes RD, et al. Incidence of and outcomes associated with ventricular tachycardia or fibrillation in patients undergoing primary percutaneous coronary intervention. JAMA 2009;301(17):1779–89.

31. Al-Khatib SM, Stevenson WG, Ackerman MJ, et al. 2017 AHA/ACC/HRS Guideline for Management of Patients With Ventricular Arrhythmias and the Prevention of Sudden Cardiac Death: A Report of the American College of Cardiology/American Heart Association Task Force on Clinical Practice Guidelines and the Hea. J Am Coll Cardiol 2018;72(14):e91–220.

32. Shaefi S, O'Gara B, Kociol RD, et al. Effect of cardiogenic shock hospital volume on mortality in patients with cardiogenic shock. J Am Heart Assoc 2015;4(1):1–9.

33. De Backer D, Biston P, Devriendt J, et al. Comparison of dopamine and norepinephrine in the treatment of shock. N Engl J Med 2010;362:779–89.

34. Alexander KP, Newby LK, Cannon CP, et al. Acute coronary care in the elderly, part I. Non-ST-segment-elevation acute coronary syndromes: A scientific

statement for healthcare professionals from the American heart association council on clinical cardiology. Circulation 2007;115(19):2549–69.

35. Kaura A, Sterne JAC, Trickey A, et al. Invasive versus non-invasive management of older patients with non-ST elevation myocardial infarction (SENIOR-NSTEMI): a cohort study based on routine clinical data. Lancet 2020;396(10251):623–34.

36. Rab T, Kern KB, Tamis-Holland JE, et al. Cardiac Arrest: A Treatment Algorithm for Emergent Invasive Cardiac Procedures in the Resuscitated Comatose Patient. J Am Coll Cardiol 2015;66(1):62–73.

37. Lemkes JS, Janssens GN, van der Hoeven NW, et al. Coronary Angiography after Cardiac Arrest without ST-Segment Elevation. N Engl J Med 2019;380(15):1397–407.

38. Abella BS, Gaieski DF. Coronary Angiography after Cardiac Arrest — The Right Timing or the Right Patients? N Engl J Med 2019;380(15):1474–5.

39. Schwartz BG, Rezkalla S, Kloner RA. Cardiovascular effects of cocaine. Circulation 2010;122(24):2558–69.

40. Mittleman MA, Mintzer D, Maclure M, et al. Triggering of myocardial infarction by cocaine. Circulation 1999;99(21):2737–41.

Medico-Legal Topics in Emergency Cardiology

John Riggins Jr, MD, Mahesh Polavarapu, MD*

KEYWORDS

- Medico-legal topics • Cardiovascular emergencies • Malpractice • Law • Risk

KEY POINTS

- Medical malpractice litigation is increasingly common in health care
- Cardiovascular chief complaints represent both present and future risks to the emergency physician.
- Eliciting and documenting key details related to a cardiovascular complaint, as well as following established standards for accurate and timely diagnosis of emergencies, is central to the medico-legal aspects of cardiovascular emergencies.
- Legal elements related to medical malpractice include the existence of a legal duty, breach of the legal duty, causation, and presence of damages.
- All 4 legal elements must be present for medical malpractice to be proven in the court of law.

INTRODUCTION

Cardiovascular complaints represent a significant volume of annual ED visits in the United States.[1] Cardiovascular emergencies are a small but noteworthy portion of these visits and can present in many ways including acute coronary syndrome, cardiac tamponade, aortic dissection, myo-endocarditis, cardiac syncope, tachy/brady arrhythmias, cardiac valvular emergencies, and cardiac arrest. Adding to the complexity of the diagnosis and management of these emergencies are the varying and overlapping symptoms with which patients can present (**Table 1**).

Furthermore, cardiovascular chief complaints pose present and future risks to the emergency physician. For example, a patient with chest pain may not be suffering from a myocardial infarction at the time of their ED evaluation but may be at high risk of an adverse cardiac event after discharge. Therefore, eliciting and documenting key details related to a cardiovascular complaint, as well as following established standards for accurate and timely diagnosis of emergencies, are central to the

Department of Emergency Medicine, Columbia University Irving Medical Center, 622 West 168th Street, VC 260, New York, NY 10032, USA
* Corresponding author.
E-mail address: Mp3921@cumc.columbia.edu

Emerg Med Clin N Am 40 (2022) 707–715
https://doi.org/10.1016/j.emc.2022.06.013
0733-8627/22/© 2022 Elsevier Inc. All rights reserved.

Table 1	
Common cardiovascular emergencies & associated chief complaints	
Acute Coronary Syndrome	chest pain/pressure, dyspnea, nausea, vomiting, diaphoresis, dizziness/lightheadedness, syncope, epigastric pain, shoulder/arm/jaw pain, generalized weakness
Cardiac Tamponade	chest pain, dyspnea, diaphoresis, lightheadedness, syncope, extremity swelling, palpitations
Aortic dissection/Aneurysm with rupture	tearing/ripping chest or back pain, sudden onset and severe, associated neurological symptoms, abdominal or flank pain, syncope
Myo-endocarditis	chest pain, fever, dyspnea, palpitations, cough, myalgias, generalized malaise, orthopnea, paroxysmal nocturnal dyspnea, abdominal pain, leg swelling, jugular venous distension
Cardiac Syncope	syncope without prodrome, preceding palpitations, chest pain, exertional dyspnea, dizziness
Tachy/Brady Arrhythmias	palpitations, dizziness/lightheadedness, chest pain/discomfort, syncope, dyspnea, nausea, vomiting, weakness
Cardiac Valvular Emergencies	exertional dyspnea, dizziness/lightheadedness, hemoptysis, orthopnea, palpitations, elevated blood pressure, low blood pressure, fatigue, chest pain
Cardiac Arrest	absence of pulses, nonperfusing cardiac rhythms

medico-legal aspects of cardiovascular emergencies. To help illustrate these principles, consider the following cases (we will revisit them throughout this article):

Case 1: A 53-year-old man with a past medical history of hypertension presents with mid-sternal chest pain. The pain woke him up from sleep, is burning, sharp, intermittent in nature, and does not migrate anywhere. He rates the pain as a 5/10, noting it gets better when he sits up and worse when he pushes on that area of his chest. He has no associated fever, chills, cough, dyspnea, dizziness, syncope, nausea, vomiting, abdominal pain, associated weakness, or numbness of his extremities. On history, he is noted to be a current smoker but denies any history of cardiac disease or stroke. Vital signs are T: 37.5 C HR: 102 BP: 160/105 RR: 16 O2 sat: 97%, and all physical exam findings are documented as normal. The emergency physician documents a differential diagnosis of acute coronary syndrome, musculoskeletal pain, pneumonia, pneumothorax, pulmonary embolism, costochondritis, peptic ulcer disease, gastritis, acute aortic dissection, and acid reflux disease. He orders an electrocardiogram (EKG), chest x –ray, and basic labs with cardiac enzymes. The EKG shows normal sinus rhythm with nonspecific T-wave changes. The chest x-ray is read as unremarkable and labs are normal, including serial negative troponins drawn four hours apart. A repeat EKG is found to have no dynamic electrocardiographic changes. Repeat vitals show T: 37.5 C HR: 88 BP: 152/90 RR: 12 O2 sat: 98%. On reassessment, the patient has no active chest pain and is discharged home with a diagnosis of musculoskeletal pain. Additionally, he is told to follow-up with his primary care doctor and the cardiology clinic and given strict return precautions to the emergency room. The patient returns the next evening complaining of severe chest pain, mid-back pain, and numbness in his right arm. After reviewing the previous visit's notes and diagnostic workup, the emergency physician orders a CT Angiogram of the chest, abdomen, and pelvis which subsequently reveals a Type A aortic dissection. The patient undergoes surgical repair, has an uneventful hospital stay, and is discharged home. The patient later files a lawsuit against the initial emergency medicine physician for failing to diagnose his dissection.

Case 2: A 61-year-old woman with a past medical history of diabetes mellitus and hypertension presents with several hours of nausea and mild left-sided chest and epigastric discomfort. The discomfort radiates to her left arm, and she had one episode of nonbloody, nonbilious emesis. Additionally, the patient notes that her symptoms started after eating clam chowder earlier in the day. She denies associated fevers, chills, cough, dyspnea, dizziness, syncope, back pain, diarrhea, hematochezia, melena, or genitourinary symptoms. She has no cardiac history, and her vitals are noted to be T: 37.4 C HR: 105 BP: 130/90 RR: 15 O2 sat: 95%. On physical exam, the emergency medicine physician documents mild epigastric discomfort but an otherwise unremarkable exam. The physician's differential diagnosis includes biliary pathology, hepatitis, pancreatitis, acute coronary syndrome, musculoskeletal pain, peptic ulcer disease, gastritis, acute aortic dissection, and acid reflux disease. An EKG, chest x-ray, comprehensive chemistry panel (including lipase and liver function tests), and cardiac enzymes are ordered. The EKG shows minimal ST-segment depressions in antero-lateral leads without reciprocal changes. The rest of the workup is unremarkable, but the patient continues to experience epigastric discomfort. The emergency medicine physician orders a right upper quadrant sonogram which shows no cholelithiasis or evidence of cholecystitis. On repeat assessment, the patient states she has some mild, persistent epigastric discomfort but overall feels better after IV fluids, ondansetron, and famotidine, and is able to tolerate oral intake of fluids. She is discharged with a diagnosis of food poisoning and acid reflux. She is instructed to follow-up with her primary care doctor but returns several hours later with worsening epigastric discomfort, chest pain, nausea, and vomiting. An EKG is performed and shows ST-segment elevations consistent with an inferior wall myocardial infarction. The cardiac catheterization lab is activated and coronary angiogram shows a right coronary artery occlusion. A drug-eluding stent is placed within the culprit vessel, but the patient develops cardiogenic shock and is sent to the Cardiac Critical Care Unit (CCU). She remains in the CCU for one month and is subsequently discharged to a subacute rehabilitation facility due to decompensation from her prolonged CCU stay. The patient brings a medical malpractice lawsuit against the first emergency medicine physician for missed diagnosis of acute myocardial infarction.

DOCUMENTATION IN CARDIOVASCULAR EMERGENCIES
History

While history taking and documentation are universally important, it is especially so in the evaluation of cardiac complaints given the present and future risk they pose. As symptoms can evolve over time, it is important to know which were present, and absent, during the time of ED evaluation. Furthermore, documenting a concise but descriptive history serves as a solid foundation for case review should litigation arise (**Box 1**).

Physical Examination

Vital signs are a key part of diagnosing and managing cardiovascular emergencies. While all vital signs should be addressed during evaluation, particular attention should

---

Box 1
Important historical features for cardiovascular emergencies

Onset of symptoms (gradual onset, sudden onset, during exertion/at rest)

Severity of symptoms (mild, moderate, severe)

Frequency and duration of symptoms (constant, intermittent, seconds/hours/days/months, and so forth)

Ameliorating and exacerbating factors (with rest, with exertion, palpation, medications, deep breathing, sitting up, laying down, worsens or improves with eating, and so forth)

Quality of pain (sharp, dull, pressure, aching, burning, and so forth)

Radiation of pain (radiates to arms, neck, jaw, back, throat, and so forth)

Location of pain (mid-chest, upper abdomen, periphery of chest, and so forth)

Associated symptoms (nausea, vomiting, dyspnea, dizziness, syncope, neck pain, arm pain, back pain, jaw pain, abdominal pain, fever, cough, neurological deficits, palpitations, hemoptysis, orthopnea, paroxysmal nocturnal dyspnea)

---

be paid to blood pressure, heart rate, and oxygen saturation (**Table 2**). One pitfall to avoid is addressing a single set of vital signs during an ED visit. Serial vital signs, including those that extend beyond the index visit, can yield valuable information.

It is also important to look for physical exam findings that can clue a provider into potential emergent/life-threatening diagnoses (**Table 3**). Should litigation arise, documentation of the presence or absence of these findings can provide insight into the

Table 2
Key vital sign abnormalities in the evaluation of cardiovascular emergencies

Abnormal Vital Sign	Things to Consider
Hypertension	• Transient hypertension in a patient can be caused by pain and/or anxiety • Attempt to compare to prior recordings, especially those from other encounters • Note if, and when, patient last took antihypertensive medications • Note responsiveness, or lack thereof, to interventions
Hypotension	• Relative hypotension compared with the patient's baseline is just as important as absolute hypotension • Attempt to compare to prior recordings, especially those from other encounters • Note if, and when, patient last took antihypertensive medications • Note responsiveness, or lack thereof, to interventions
Tachycardia	• May represent serious underlying etiology such as tachyarrhythmia, hypovolemia, shock, ischemia, or toxic metabolic derangements • Could be secondary to pain, fever, or anxiety
Bradycardia	• May represent serious underlying etiology such as hypoglycemia, hypoxia, metabolic derangement, toxidrome, or heart block • May represent a benign cause such as increased vagal tone, athleticism, or drug side effect and therapeutic dose (beta-blockers, calcium channel blockers, and so forth)
Hypoxia	• Consider severe anemia, V/Q mismatch, underlying congenital cardiac abnormalities, shock, and toxidromes • Ensure patient's baseline oxygen requirements are met

provider's thought process and medical decision making. Care should be taken when documenting a normal exam using macros that might be provided in the electronic medical record. For example, if a patient is noted to be tachycardic on initial vitals and remains tachycardic on physical exam, one should ensure "tachycardic" is documented in the cardiac portion of the exam. One should also remember to only document portions of the physical exam that are performed, keeping in mind that a full physical exam is not always required in the emergency department.

Relation to case 1: The medical provider documented the physical examination as normal and addressed the initial abnormal vital signs. The provider also appropriately repeated the physical examination and looked for any evolution in exam findings that could change diagnostic work-up or disposition.

Relation to case 2: The medical provider documented an appropriate physical exam with relevant abnormalities (epigastric pain noted upon the palpation of the abdomen). The medical provider also conducted a repeat focused exam, reassessed the patient's pain, and performed a PO challenge prior to discharge in the setting of a suspected abdominal complaint and GI diagnosis. However, the provider failed to address and recheck the patient's abnormal vital signs (tachycardia noted during initial vitals). While normal vital signs are not a prerequisite for ED discharge, one should comment on persistent vital sign abnormalities. This includes thorough the documentation of what may be driving abnormal vital signs, the lack of indication for further observation and/or admission, and follow-up and/or return precautions discussed with the patient regarding such findings.

Diagnostic Work-Up and Medical Decision Making

Diagnostic modalities for the evaluation of cardiac complaints are not only extensive, but vary from cheap, minimally invasive, and harmless, to costly, invasive, and associated with harm. Therefore, workups should be tailored to the diagnoses being considered. The medical provider should perform due diligence in incorporating the results of these diagnostic workups into their medical decision making (**Box 2**).

MEDICAL LAW AND MEDICAL MALPRACTICE

Medical law, as defined by the Institute of Medicine and Law, constitutes the responsibilities of medical professionals and the rights of patients. These rights and responsibilities center on confidentiality, criminal law, ethics, and torts.[2] The most familiar form of tort related to medical law is medical malpractice which will be the focus of this article. However, it is important to recognize that other forms of tort exist. For example, performing treatment on a patient who declines such treatment can constitute battery and wrongfully disclosing information about a patient's health can constitute defamation.

Table 3	
Key physical examination findings in cardiovascular emergencies	
Mental Status	**Jugular Venous Distension**
Presence of wheezes/rales/rhonchi	Presence of S3/S4 gallop
Pulse Asymmetry	Focal Neurological Deficits
Presence of murmur	Muffled Heart Sounds
Cyanosis	Presence of Janeway lesions/Osler Nodes
Presence of Pedal Edema	Abdominal Tenderness/Distension

Box 2
Common diagnostic modalities for cardiac complaints

Electrocardiogram to look for ischemic changes, evidence of ST-elevation MI, tachy/brady arrhythmias, and other concerning EKG patterns

Chest X-ray to look for signs of widened mediastinum, fluid overload, infection, pneumothorax, surgical interventions

Bedside ultrasound to evaluate for pericardial effusion, ejection fraction, thrombus, dissection flap, presence of aneurysm

Basic metabolic panel to assess for electrolyte abnormalities, kidney function

Complete blood count to assess for leukopenia/leukocytosis, anemia/polycythemia, thrombocytosis/thrombocytopenia

Cardiac enzymes to assess for myocardial injury

CT angiogram chest/abdomen/pelvis to assess for dissection, aneurysm, intramural thrombus

---

Medical malpractice pertains to a medical professional's liability for negligence in the diagnosis or treatment of a patient that directly results in injury or death[2] Negligence is further defined as "the standard of conduct to which one must conform… [and] is that of a reasonable man under like circumstances."[3–5] Medical malpractice lawsuits are increasingly common in health care, with an estimated 75% of health care providers in low-risk specialties and 99% in high-risk specialties facing a lawsuit by the age of 65.[6] It is important to note that a lawsuit alleging medical malpractice must be filed within a specified period set by the state for which the case is filed. This period is called the "statute of limitations" and a case filed outside of it will be dismissed. In the United States, unlike many other countries, medical malpractice suits traditionally fall under the jurisdiction of individual states and not the federal government. A common exception to this rule is when care is provided through a federally funded source or a Veteran's Administration (VA) facility, in which case action is taken through a federal district court.

Given the common occurrence of medical malpractice lawsuits and the associated risk of financial damages being rewarded, most medical providers in the United States carry malpractice insurance. However, it is important to note that malpractice cases rarely go to trial. Rather, the legal system is built to promote self-resolution through the process of discovery and other legal tools. When a case does go to trial, 4 key elements are required to successfully prove medical negligence in the court of law. All 4 legal elements must be present for medical malpractice to be proven. A plaintiff will work to gather proof through the collection of medical records, expert testimony, reviewing prior malpractice claims, and creation of a timeline of events. These 4 key elements are:

Existence of a legal duty

The first legal element that must be proven by the defendant is the existence of a professional relationship between the physician and the patient. If such relationship does not exist, there is no legal duty presumed. A professional relationship between physician and patient is created when a physician takes ownership of the patient's care. This can also be applied to covering for a colleague's patient and consulting for a patient as a specialist. Once a professional relationship is established, a reasonable duty of care is expected. In the emergency room setting, as in most health care settings, this legal element is the easiest to establish.

Relation to case 1 and case 2: The initial emergency medicine physician in each case took care of the patient, thereby establishing a professional relationship between physician and patient. As this professional relationship existed, a legal duty to the patient was presumed and reasonable duty of care was expected.

Breach of the legal duty

The second element that must be proven by the plaintiff is that there was a breach of the physician's legal duty to provide reasonable care, also called standard of care, to the patient. Standard of care is defined as "…not a guideline or list of options; instead, it is a duty determined by a given set of circumstances that present in a particular patient, with a specific condition, at a definite time and place."[7,8] In other words, if placed in the same scenario with the same patient, would the majority of emergency medicine physicians' medical decision making be the same or comparable to that of the physician in question, and would their actions fall in line with those made by a said physician? This legal element usually requires an expert witness to evaluate appropriate standards of care in a medico-legal case.

Relation to case 1: The plaintiff argued that as aortic dissection was on the list of differential diagnoses for chest pain, not ordering a CT Angiogram represented a breach of legal duty to provide reasonable care. The defendant argued that physician documentation noted a normal physical exam, including symmetrical pulses throughout, and the absence of neurological deficits. Furthermore, the pain was not severe or sudden in onset and did not radiate to the back or abdomen. ED workup, which included chest radiography, was normal. As aortic dissection was one of the many potential diagnoses on the differential, not ordering a CT Angiogram did not violate the established standard of care for patients presenting with chest pain.

Relation to case 2: The plaintiff argued that the standard of care was not met because the emergency medicine physician failed to order serial EKG and serial cardiac enzymes to evaluate for acute myocardial infarction in a patient with persistent pain. The plaintiff also argued that the emergency provider failed to repeat and reassess abnormal vital signs. Lastly, clear, and precise, return precautions were not provided to the patient at the time of discharge from the ED. The defendant argued that the emergency medicine physician's history and physical exam were consistent with a gastrointestinal (GI) etiology and the emergency medicine physician appropriately ordered abdominal imaging, EKG, and chemistry panel to rule out life-threatening emergencies. The defendant also argued that the patient's symptoms were reassessed, and acceptable discharge parameters for acute GI illness were met prior to ED discharge. Lastly, the defendant noted that appropriate instructions to follow-up with a primary care doctor were given.

Causation

Although there may be a deviation from the standard of care in a medico-legal complaint, there is no legal case of negligence unless the deviation can be factually attributed to direct patient harm. If direct harm due to deviation from standard of care cannot be shown within reason of medical certainty, negligence cannot be proven in the court of law. In contrast to the legal duty, this element of medical malpractice is usually the most difficult to establish.

Relation to case 1: The plaintiff argued that the delay in diagnosis of an acute aortic dissection led to pain, suffering and a prolonged hospital stay for the patient. The defendant argued that the patient was cared for appropriately during the first medical encounter and the delay in diagnosis of an acute aortic dissection was not directly related to any actions taken by the initial ED provider given the history, physical exam, and diagnostic findings. Furthermore, the defendant argued that symptoms present during the second visit could have been distinct and separate from those during the initial encounter; and the acute aortic dissection could have developed after the patient was discharged from the emergency department. Therefore, causation could not be proven within reason of medical certainty.

Relation to case 2: The plaintiff argued that failure to obtain repeat EKG and serial cardiac enzymes led to a delayed diagnosis of acute myocardial infarction. This subsequently caused irreversible damage to the patient's heart, prolonged hospitalization, and a prolonged subacute rehabilitation stay. The defendant argued that the patient's initial visit was deemed more consistent with a gastrointestinal diagnosis and the acute myocardial infarction could have developed after the patient went home. Furthermore, cardiogenic shock is a known complication of inferior wall myocardial infarction. This complication, and its downstream effects, could have been independent of any potential delay in diagnosis during the initial ED visit.

Presence of damages

The fourth key element needed to prove medical malpractice is the presence of damages. If no damages occur due to the alleged negligence, medical malpractice cannot be proven in court. Damages are calculated as compensatory or punitive. Compensatory damages are, as the name implies, meant to compensate for things such as medical bills, wages lost, and pain and suffering incurred. Punitive damages are rarely a part of medical malpractice litigation and are reserved mostly for heinous acts such as sexual misconduct.

Relation to case 1: There were no lasting damages to the patient.

Relation to case 2: Compensatory damages were present and included significant medical expenses, prolonged hospital and subacute rehabilitation stays, and lost wages from being unable to work for an extended period. No punitive damages were present.

SUMMARY

Case 1 determination: It was deemed that the physician performed and documented a thorough history and physical exam. Diagnostic workup was appropriately ordered and interpreted. His vital signs were repeated, showing the resolution of tachycardia, and a repeat EKG showed no dynamic changes. The patient was reassessed and had no pain at the time of discharge. The patient was discharged with strict return precautions and appropriate outpatient follow-up. While the diagnosis of aortic dissection may have been missed, the emergency medicine physician was not found to have breached his legal duty to the patient, and there were no lasting damages. The case was, therefore, adjudicated in favor of the defendant.

Case 2 determination: Although the emergency medicine physician ordered an EKG, chest x-ray, and cardiac enzymes, the physician failed to repeat an abnormal EKG to assess for dynamic changes in a patient with persistent pain. The physician also failed to reassess abnormal vital signs before discharge. The diagnostic workup was felt to have deviated from accepted standards as no repeat cardiac enzyme testing was performed and the abnormal EKG was not addressed. Lastly, clear return precautions were not given to the patient at the time of discharge. As such, all 4 legal elements were deemed met. The emergency medicine physician had a legal duty to the patient given the established professional relationship. There was a breach of this duty as deviation from standard practice was present. This breach led to a delayed diagnosis of acute myocardial infarction and subsequent compensatory damages (cardiogenic shock, prolonged hospitalization, high hospital costs, subacute rehabilitation stay, subacute rehabilitation costs, and loss of wages). The case was adjudicated in favor of the plaintiff.

One key takeaway from these illustrative cases is that while it may not be possible to eliminate risk when assessing for cardiovascular emergencies, risk can certainly be mitigated.

CLINICS CARE POINTS

- Elicit and document key historical details and physical exam findings
- Make sure to address all complaints in the documented "chief complaint"
- Document and address any relevant vital sign, electrocardiogram (EKG), lab, or imaging abnormalities during the patient's work-up
- Medical decision making should include a differential diagnosis instead of a restatement of the workup being conducted.
- Document any refusal of care by the patient in your chart and his/her rationale for the refusal of care
- Use professionally accepted algorithms to justify diagnostic testing and disposition of the patient
- Give clear and concise discharge instructions to the patient
- Ensure that the patient has appropriate outpatient follow up

DISCLOSURES

The authors have nothing to disclose.

REFERENCES

1. Anjum S. Systematic approach to acute cardiovascular emergencies. Essentials Accid Emerg Med 2019;193–228. https://doi.org/10.5772/intechopen.71634.
2. Hg.org Legal Resources. Medical Law. Available at: https://www.hg.org/medical-law.html. Accessed January 31, 2022.
3. Moffett P, Moore G. The standard of care: legal history and definitions: the bad and good news. West J Emerg Med 2011;12(1):109–12.
4. Bal BS. An introduction to medical malpractice in the United States. Clin Orthop Relat Res 2009;467(2):339–47.
5. Gittler GJ, Goldstein EJC. The elements of medical malpractice: an overview. Clin Infect Dis 1996;23(5):1152–5.
6. Jena AB, Seabury S, Lakdawalla D, et al. Malpractice risk according to physician specialty. N Engl J Med 2011;365(7):629–36.
7. Grady A. The importance of standard of care and documentation. Virtual Mentor 2005;7(11):756–8.
8. Ferguson B, Geralds J, Petrey J, et al. Malpractice in emergency medicine-a review of risk and mitigation practices for the emergency medicine provider. J Emerg Med 2018;55(5):659–65.

Narrow Complex Tachycardias

Tareq Al-Salamah, MBBS, MPH[a,b,*], Mohammed AlAgeel, MBBS[a,c,1],
Leen Alblaihed, MBBS, MHA[b]

KEYWORDS

- Narrow-complex tachycardia • Supraventricular tachycardia • Tachydysrhythmia
- Tachycardia

KEY POINTS

- The differential diagnosis for commonly encountered narrow complex tachycardias in the emergency department is limited.
- A good understanding of the pathophysiology behind the different types of narrow complex tachycardias is key to making the diagnosis and understanding management options.
- Scrutiny of the electrocardiogram can yield subtle findings that can reveal the diagnosis and significantly alter management options.
- Narrow complex tachycardias can occur as a result of or as a result of a presenting condition.

NARROW COMPLEX TACHYCARDIAS

Introduction

Palpitations are a common presenting symptom to the emergency department (ED), accounting for over 50,000 annual visits in the United States, with often benign underlying etiologies.[1] Underlying cardiac etiologies are identified in 34% to 43% of these presentations.[1,2] The prevalence of supraventricular tachycardias (SVT) in the general population is thought to be 2.29 per 1000 people.[3]

Tachydysrhythmias range from benign to malignant rhythms. Emergency physicians must be able to accurately diagnose these conditions to deliver appropriate and timely interventions to prevent potential deleterious complications, as some forms

[a] Department of Emergency Medicine, King Saud University, College of Medicine, PO Box 7805, Riyadh 11472, Saudi Arabia; [b] Department of Emergency Medicine, University of Maryland, School of Medicine, Baltimore, MD, USA; [c] Department of Emergency Medicine, University of British Columbia, Vancouver, British Columbia, Canada
[1] Present address: PO Box 250938, Riyadh 11391.
* Corresponding author.
E-mail address: tareq.salamah@gmail.com
Twitter: @SalamahTareq (T.A.-S.); @AgeelMoe (M.A.)

Emerg Med Clin N Am 40 (2022) 717–732
https://doi.org/10.1016/j.emc.2022.06.009
0733-8627/22/© 2022 Elsevier Inc. All rights reserved.

of tachycardia, if untreated, can lead to stroke, heart failure (ie, tachycardia-induced cardiomyopathy), cardiovascular collapse, and death.

Pathophysiology

Narrow refers to a QRS complex duration of less than 120 milliseconds, or three small boxes on an electrocardiogram (ECG), and tachycardia is defined as a rate greater than 100 beats per minute (bpm). Tachycardia originating at, or above, the level of the His–Purkinje bundle is termed SVT. When ventricular depolarization is propagated normally through the bundle branches and ventricular myocardium, SVT gives rise to a narrow complex tachycardia (NCT). NCTs are commonly seen on 12-lead ECG recordings of patients in the ED.

Wide complex tachycardias (WCT) develop when the rhythm originates below the His–Purkinje bundle, termed "ventricular tachycardia" (VT), or when an SVT propagates abnormally through the ventricles (eg, fixed or rate-related bundle branch blocks, metabolic abnormalities, sodium channel blocker toxicity, and so forth).

Tachydysrhythmias are thought to occur through one of three mechanisms: reentry, triggered activity, or problems with automaticity.

Re-entrant tachycardias require a trigger, such as premature depolarization in the form of a premature atrial complex (PAC) or premature ventricular complex, and a substrate to initiate and sustain the arrhythmia, respectively. The substrate is "a loop" or two connected pathways (eg, scar or fibrosis from prior myocardial infarction, surgery, or cardiomyopathy) that differ in conduction speed and refractoriness. Usually, one pathway has fast conduction with a long refractory period, and the other has slow conduction with a short refractory period (**Fig. 1**).

Triggered activity results from the premature activation of the cardiac cells by an afterdepolarization. In other words, it occurs when a new depolarization occurs during or after the repolarization phase. Early afterdepolarizations (EAD) occur during phase 2 or 3 of the cardiac action potential during the repolarization phase due to the opening of L-type calcium channels. Prolonged QT interval, bradycardia, hypokalemia, acidosis, and hypoxia can cause EAD. Delayed afterdepolarizations (DAD) occur after the full repolarization phase (phase 4 of the action potential) and are due to intracellular calcium overload. Ischemia, hypercalcemia, and digoxin toxicity can cause DAD.

Automaticity can be either enhanced or abnormal. Enhanced automaticity describes when a normal automatic focus [eg, sinoatrial (SA) node] shows enhanced automaticity (eg, inappropriate sinus tachycardia). Abnormal automaticity describes when pacing is from a focus that is not considered a normal automatic focus (eg, an ectopic atrial focus in focal atrial tachycardia).

DISCUSSION
Approach to Tachydysrhythmias

A reasonable approach to diagnosing the type of tachydysrhythmias is to obtain a quality ECG and assess the QRS complex duration (<120 milliseconds is narrow, ≥120 milliseconds is wide) and the rhythm (regular or irregular based on the RR interval). This initial categorization can help narrow the differential diagnosis and help guide management.

Regular, narrow complex tachycardias

Commonly encountered differential diagnoses in the ED for regular NCT include sinus tachycardia, atrial flutter (AFL) with fixed conduction, atrioventricular nodal re-entrant tachycardia (AVNRT), and orthodromic atrioventricular re-entrant tachycardia. **Table 1**

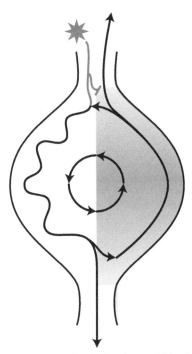

Fig. 1. Re-entrant circuit: A re-entrant circuit develops within tissue containing two pathways for impulses to travel through; a "slow" pathway with a short (ie, fast) refractory period (referred to as the "slow-fast" pathway), and a "fast" pathway with a long (ie, slow) refractory period (referred to as the "fast-slow" pathway).[4] (Figure courtesy of Dr. AbdulAziz AlKanhal)

features ECG findings and some diagnostic hints for the most commonly encountered regular NCTs.

1. *Sinus tachycardia* occurs due to enhanced automaticity from the SA node. It is the most common tachycardia as it is a normal response to physiologic or pathologic stressors, or to sympathomimetics and some drugs. Heart rate ranges between 100 and 220. On ECG, sinus P-waves are upright in leads I, II, and aVF, biphasic in lead V1, and usually inverted in aVR (**Figs. 2** and **3**).
2. *Sinus node re-entry tachycardia* is a pathological tachydysrhythmia caused by a re-entrant circuit in the SA node. The ECG recording appears identical to sinus tachycardia; patients often report an abrupt onset and termination of palpitations.
3. *Focal atrial tachycardia* is commonly due to a single focus with increased automaticity in a normal atrium or less commonly, a re-entry circuit in diseased or scarred atrial tissue.[5] It is often instigated by increased catecholamine states. Rates range between 150 and <250 bpm, and the P-wave axis depends on the location of this focus. See **Fig. 4**. Patients usually present with palpitations, shortness of breath, or chest pain. Rarely do patients present with syncope or presyncope.

There is limited evidence to suggest the best treatment approach for atrial tachycardia. Generally, beta-blockers and calcium channel blockers (CCB) may convert back to sinus rhythm or slow the ventricular rate. Synchronized cardioversion often terminates focal atrial tachycardia. For recurrent or incessant forms, catheter ablation is the treatment of choice.

Table 1
Features of often encountered regular NCTs in the ED

| | Sinus Tachycardia | Atrial Flutter (with 2:1 or 3:1 AVN Conduction) | Re-entry Circuit with AVN Involvement | |
			AVNRT	Orthodromic AVRT
Ventricular rate range bpm (Avg)	100 to (age − 220)	130–170 bpm (150) 2:1 conduction (atrial rate 250–330 bpm)	110–250 bpm	140–280 bpm
ECG features	Regular rhythm, with normal[a] P-waves for every QRS Variation in rate	Sawtooth pattern Regular rhythm, and often abnormal[b] P-waves with one morphology More P-waves than QRS complexes	Regular QRS complexes with absent (buried) or retrograde P-waves for every QRS complex	
Diagnostic hints/suggestions	Clinical condition and presentation usually allude to an underlying cause for sinus tachycardia	Sawtooth pattern on ECG with inverted (most common) P-waves in inferior leads, and upright P-waves in V1. Minimally-fluctuating (fixed) ventricular rate on the monitor Notching within QRS complexes or T-waves when P-waves are noted between two QRS complexes or between two T-waves (Bix rule)	Rapid rates than would be expected for sinus tachycardia and atrial flutter with absent P-waves Rapid on and off	

Abbreviations: AC, anticoagulation; AF, atrial fibrillation; AFL, atrial flutter; AP, accessory pathway; AVN, atrioventricular node; AVNRT, atrioventricular nodal re-entrant tachycardia; AVRT, atrioventricular re-entrant tachycardia; Bpm, beats per minute; ECG, electrocardiogram.
[a] Normal P-waves refer to sinus P-waves similar to prior baseline ECGs.
[b] Abnormal P-waves include retrograde P-waves or P-waves with a morphology that differs from that found in prior baseline ECGs.

4. *Junctional tachycardia* is an uncommon tachydysrhythmia that arises within the AVN or proximal His–Purkinje bundle due to enhanced automaticity. It usually occurs in children following cardiac procedures or surgery. It is also seen in ischemia, stimulant, or digitalis toxicity. ECG recordings usually show a NCT at a rate from 100 to 130 bpm and retrograde P-waves. Treatment is directed at the underlying cause or toxicity.[6]

5. *AFL* is a supraventricular re-entrant tachydysrhythmia with the re-entry loop (circuit) just above the AVN in the right atrium. The loop usually runs in a counterclockwise direction (90%), producing the "typical" classic negative (sawtooth) flutter waves in the inferior leads (II, III, aVF).[7] See **Fig. 5**. It is the second most common sustained pathological arrhythmia after atrial fibrillation (AF).[7] A less common

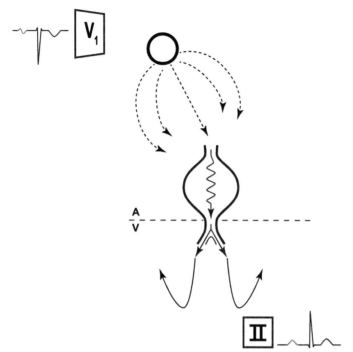

Fig. 2. Sinus tachycardia: electrical impulse originates from the SA node, travels through the atrial myocardium (*dashed arrows*) toward the atrioventricular node (AVN), travels through the AVN at a slower conduction rate (*wavy arrow*), then travels rapidly down the His–Purkinje system to the ventricular myocardium (*solid arrows*). The ECG shows a biphasic P-wave (*dashed*) in lead V1 because of the electrical impulse initially traveling toward, then away from V1, as it travels through the left atrium, whereas lead II shows upright P-waves (*dashed*) due to the electrical impulse traveling toward it. (Figure courtesy of Dr. AbdulAziz AlKanhal)

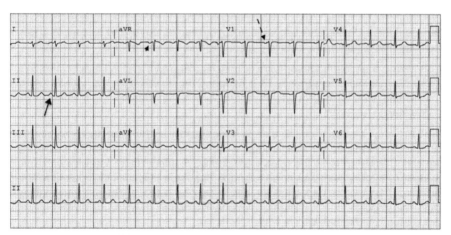

Fig. 3. Sinus tachycardia: In this ECG, the atrial and ventricular rates are 104 bpm, and every QRS complex is preceded by a "normal" P-wave (ie, biphasic in lead V1 (*dashed arrow*), upright in inferior leads (*solid arrow*), and inverted in aVR (*arrow head*)), suggesting the atrial electrical impulse is originating from the SA node. (ECG courtesy of Dr. Ahmed B AlSalem)

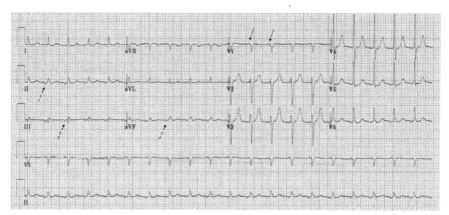

Fig. 4. Focal Atrial Tachycardia: In this ECG, atrial and ventricular beats are at a rate of 120 bpm. The atrial electrical impulses are traveling toward the area of the SA node (identified by P-waves upright in V1 (*solid arrow*) and inverted in the inferior leads (*dashed arrows*)), suggesting an ectopic atrial focus. AFL is less likely because the atrial rate is below the flutter range of 250–330 bpm. The differential diagnoses also include atypical AVNRT and junctional tachycardia. (Source: https://litfl.com/atrial-tachycardia-ecg-library/)

variant known as "reverse typical" is characterized by upright flutter waves in the inferior leads due to clockwise movement of the circuit. The location of the circuit is around the tricuspid annulus (cavotricuspid isthmus) in the right atrium, with the classification of AFL based on the direction of the re-entry loop.

The rhythm is generated by a re-entrant circuit producing a regular, rapid atrial rate of 250–300 bmp. However, the healthy AVN will slow down impulse conduction to the ventricles and will not conduct all the impulses. The ventricular rate is some fraction of the atrial rate (fixed 2:1, 3:1 atrial:ventricular rate) and usually does not exceed 200 bmp, unless an accessory pathway (AP) exists bypassing the AVN. A higher degree of block is seen in patients on AV nodal blockers or if the AVN is diseased.[7] Additionally, AFL can present as an irregular rhythm due to variable AVN conduction.

Aside from a notable male predominance, causes, risk factors, presentation, and management, including anticoagulation (AC), are similar to AF and discussed in detail later (see discussion on AF below).[8]

6. *AVNRT* is the most common form of nonsustained SVT and the most common tachydysrhythmia in pregnancy.[3,9] It happens most often in young adults without structural heart disease or prior myocardial insult (eg, infarction), with a female predominance (>63%).[9]

AVNRT is a re-entrant circuit that develops within an AV node that contains two pathways for impulses to travel through; a "slow" pathway with a short (ie, fast) refractory period (referred to as the "slow-fast' pathway), and a "fast" pathway with a long (ie, slow) refractory period (referred to as the "fast-slow" pathway).[4] A perfectly timed and located premature depolarization can instigate the circuit. The pathway that conducts the impulse in an anterograde manner dictates the type of AVNRT (typical versus atypical) (**Figs. 6–8**).

AVNRT commonly occurs spontaneously but can also be provoked with stimulants or alcohol. Patients commonly present with palpitations, dizziness, and/or shortness of breath.[10,11] AVNRT is rarely life-threatening, and although syncope is not common, it tends to occur in patients over 65 years of age.[10,12]

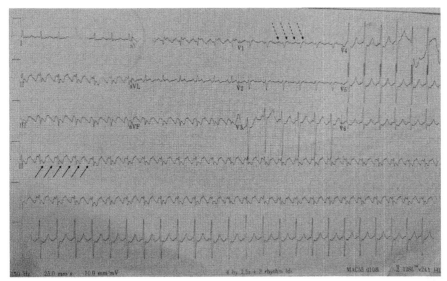

Fig. 5. AFL: This is AFL with 2:1 atrial:ventricular conduction. This ECG demonstrates AFL's classic "Sawtooth" pattern created by the inverted flutter waves in the inferior leads (II, III, and aVF) (*solid arrows*). Note the upright flutter waves in lead V1 (*dashed arrows*), suggesting an ectopic origin of atrial electrical activity.

7. *AVRT* is the second most common form of nonsustained SVT; it is a re-entrant tachydysrhythmia with the circuit consisting of the AVN (slow conduction and short refractory period) and an AP bypassing the AVN connecting the atria to the ventricles (with fast conduction and long refractory period). It is classified into orthodromic and antidromic based on the direction of conduction through the AVN.

Orthodromic AVRT accounts for 90–95% of SVT occurring in patients with an AP and refers to electrical impulses traveling anterogradely through the AVN toward the ventricles, then retrograde through the AP to the atria (**Fig. 9**). Ventricular rates in orthodromic AVRT range between 140 and 280 bpm,[13] and rarely exceed 220 bpm.[6] ECG findings are similar to those in atypical AVNRT with narrow QRS complexes (<120 milliseconds) and, if apparent and not buried, retrograde P-waves show up inverted in the inferior leads and upright in lead V1, often just before the following QRS complex.

Antidromic AVRT is much less common than orthodromic AVRT and accounts for 5% of SVT in patients with an AP. Electrical impulses travel in the opposite direction of that in orthodromic AVRT, where ventricular depolarization begins at the connection site of the AP, resulting in a regular *WCT*. Although treatment is similar to that of orthodromic AVRT, differentiating it from VT can be very challenging in the ED setting (**Fig. 10**). This topic is covered in detail in the "Wide Complex Tachycardia" article in this series of EMClinics.

Treatment of narrow complex, regular rhythm tachycardias

Treatment depends on the diagnosis and the patient's clinical condition. As sinus tachycardia is a response to a physiologic or pathologic process, management should be directed toward correcting the underlying cause. Treatment of AFL follows that of AF (detailed under "Special considerations in the treatment of atrial fibrillation and atrial flutter" below).

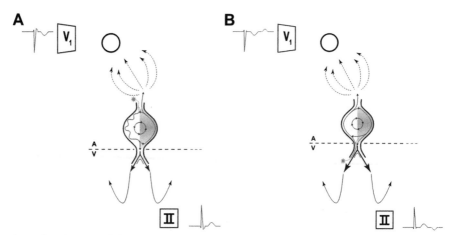

Fig. 6. (*A, B*) AVNRT: (*A*) Typical AVNRT occurs when a premature atrial depolarization (*star*) enters this circuit and travels as depicted in the image. The P-wave (*dashed tracing*), if not fully buried, is retrograde (inverted in inferior leads and upright in V1) and will be just preceding or following the QRS complex (short R-P interval), noted at the terminal part of the S-wave (*dashed tracing*) in this figure, giving rise to the "pseudo-S wave." (*B*) The atypical AVNRT mechanism is similar but is instigated by a premature ventricular depolarization (*star*) and enters the circuit from below in the opposite direction of that in typical AVNRT. Note the retrograde P-waves (as in typical AVNRT) but at a longer distance (long RP interval) from the QRS complex, sometimes appearing prior to the following QRS complex. (Figures courtesy of Dr. AbdulAziz AlKanhal)

We now provide a detailed discussion on treatment options for paroxysmal SVT (ie, AVNRT and AVRT).

The goal of treatment in paroxysmal SVT is to disrupt the re-entrant circuit by altering conduction through the AVN because it is a part of the circuit in both AVNRT and AVRT. This can be done with vagal maneuvers (via activating baroreceptors), medications (such as adenosine, CCB, and beta-blockers), or with electrical cardioversion. Synchronized electrical cardioversion is the fastest method to break the circuit and restore sinus rhythm, but due to the associated pain and discomfort, synchronized electrical cardioversion is recommended as first-line in patients with hemodynamic instability or as a last option in the ED after failure of vagal maneuvers and medications. Start at 50–100 J, then double if the first dose fails.

Vagal maneuvers, such as the Valsalva maneuver, modified Valsalva, carotid sinus massage, and diver reflex, are first line before advancing to medications in stable

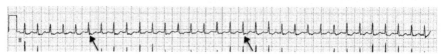

Fig. 7. Typical AVNRT: In this lead II rhythm strip, the ventricles are beating at a rate of 192 bpm, with regular, narrow QRS complexes and retrograde P-waves immediately following QRS complexes. Inverted P-waves are noted (*arrows*) right after the QRS complexes (short RP interval; P-wave close to R-wave), giving rise to apparent "deep S-waves." The differential diagnosis here includes an arrhythmia with a circuit reentry involving the AVN [typical AVNRT, orthodromic atrioventricular reciprocating tachycardia (AVRT)], and junctional tachycardia (although less likely given the rapid rate on this ECG).

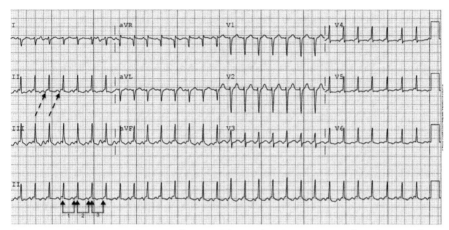

Fig. 8. Atypical AVNRT: In this ECG, the ventricles are beating at a rate of 178 bpm, with regular, narrow QRS complexes, and retrograde P-waves are noted inverted in inferior leads (*dashed arrows*) and far from the QRS complexes (long RP interval). Note the *grouped solid arrows* are numbered to represent QRS and atrial beats that belong together. The differential diagnosis here includes an arrhythmia with a circuit re-entry involving the AVN (atypical AVNRT, orthodromic AVRT) and atrial tachycardia. (ECG courtesy of Dr. Ahmed B AlSalem)

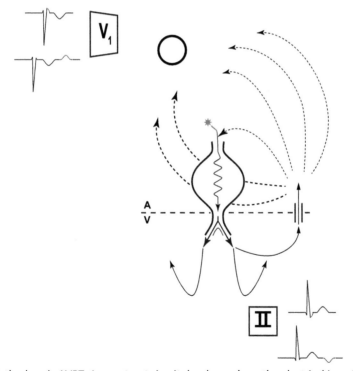

Fig. 9. Orthodromic AVRT: A re-entrant circuit develops where the electrical impulse travels from the atria (*dashed arrows*) through the AVN, down the His–Purkinje system anterogradely spreading through the ventricles (*solid arrows*), then back to the atria retrogradely through an AP. The P-wave on ECG has similar features to AVNRT and can be difficult to differentiate. (Figure courtesy of Dr. AbdulAziz AlKanhal)

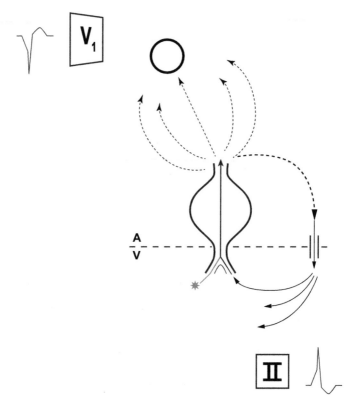

Fig. 10. Antidromic AVRT: A re-entrant circuit develops where the electrical impulse travels from the ventricles (*solid arrows*) through the AVN, retrogradely spreading through the atria (*dashed arrows*), then back to the ventricles anterogradely through an AP. Note that QRS complexes are wide due to ventricular depolarization through the AP. (Figure courtesy of Dr. AbdulAziz AlKanhal)

patients due to their ease, low cost, association with minimal risk, and have been found to terminate paroxysmal SVT with success up to 50% of cases.[14] The easiest and most recognized of which is the "Valsalva maneuver" which entails lying in a supine position while straining against resistance (such as a closed glottis) for 15 to 30 seconds with the goal of increasing intrathoracic pressure.[15] A modified version of the Valsalva has been studied in the "REVERT trial" and validated by Corbacioglu and colleagues[16,17] and showed a higher success rate in comparison with the original Valsalva maneuver (10%–17% versus over 42%). The modified version entails the patient blowing against a resistance of 40 mm Hg sustained for 15 seconds while sitting in a semirecumbent position then immediately lying flat and having the care team raise the patient's legs to 15°–45° degrees.

Of the medications that alter conduction through the AVN, adenosine, CCB, and beta-blockers are recommended in that respective order in the 2015 AHA and 2019 ESC Guidelines on the management of patients with SVT.[6,13]

Despite similar efficacy rates (over 90%) in reverting SVT to sinus rhythm, adenosine is recommended as first line (along with vagal maneuvers) in the most recent American and European Guidelines.[18,19] Data on beta-blockers are lacking and recommendations for their use are restricted to cases of failed reversion after adenosine and

CCB, or when CCB is contraindicated. Care must be taken to factor in potential contraindications to the respective drugs, which further guides the choice of drug.

Furthermore, adenosine and vagal maneuvers can be used to differentiate SVT from AFL. In AFL, the AVN is not involved in the flutter circuit and thus will not be terminated by adenosine or vagal maneuvers which can unmask flutter waves.

In pregnant patients, initial treatment of SVT is similar to that of nonpregnant patients, with some precautions to be kept in mind. Synchronized electrical cardioversion is recommended in hemodynamically compromised patients as first line in the European Guidelines, followed by vagal maneuvers and then adenosine. In the 2015 AHA/ACC guidelines, the recommendation is to start with vagal maneuvers followed by adenosine in unstable patients, then synchronized electrical cardioversion if adenosine fails. Vagal maneuvers are very low risk and may obviate the need to use medications or electrical cardioversion. Adenosine is considered safe in pregnancy. Although the risk to the fetus is low with electrical cardioversion, fetal and toco-monitoring are recommended. In the event of their failure, the guidelines support the use of beta-blockers before CCB due to their safety profile in pregnant women. If beta-blockers fail and CCB are considered, then verapamil is recommended over diltiazem.[6,13]

Irregular, narrow complex tachycardias

As the name implies, these tachycardias present with narrow QRS complexes and irregular RR intervals on ECG. The irregularity in narrow complex ventricular beats results from irregular atrial electrical impulses [eg, AF, multifocal atrial tachycardia (MAT), frequent PACs], or variable conduction of regular atrial impulses (eg, AFL with variable conduction).

1. *MAT* is an uncommon irregular tachydysrhythmia defined by the presence of ≥3 distinct P-wave morphologies in the same lead on ECG, representing ≥3 atrial foci, and variable PP, PR, and RR intervals, and a distinct isoelectric line between P-waves The underlying pathophysiology is not clear and may be due to enhanced automaticity, triggering, or re-entry. It is often an incidental rhythm found in an asymptomatic patient with chronic cardiopulmonary disease and electrolyte abnormalities.[20] **Fig. 11**. Most cases of MAT do not lead to hemodynamic compromise, and treatment is based on managing the underlying disease rather than the arrhythmia.

2. *Premature atrial and junctional complexes (PACs and PJCs)* are premature activation of the atria from a site other than the SA node, within the atria in PACs, and near the atrioventricular junction in PJCs. On ECG, PACs yield a P-wave morphology and a PR interval that differ from baseline due to the nonsinus origin of the depolarizations. P-waves in PJCs are often absent or retrograde on ECG. The frequency of PACs and PJCs can vary from occasional to very frequent, up to every other sinus beat (ie, atrial bigeminy), producing a regularly irregular NCT. PACs and PJCs are usually benign and do not require treatment in the ED.

3. *AFL with variable conduction* presents with an irregular rate due to conduction of atrial impulses through the AVN at variable ratios. ECG findings are similar to those mentioned in AFL earlier except for variable RR intervals alternating among 2:1, 3:1, and 4:1 conduction ratios.

4. *AF* is the most common sustained pathological arrhythmia seen in the ED, characterized by a disorganized, rapid, and irregular atrial rhythm with an often rapid ventricular response. It can be a primary disease due to structural changes in the heart or secondary due to an acute medical condition. The duration is classified as

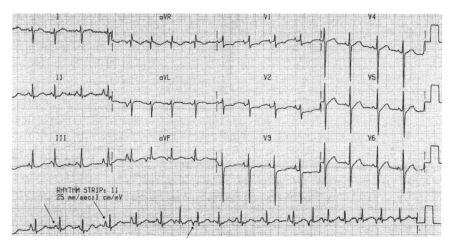

Fig. 11. MAT: In this ECG, there is a tachycardia at a rate of 108 bpm and an irregular rhythm with ≥3 P-wave morphologies in the same lead (*arrows*) representing multiple atrial beats from multiple atrial foci, with irregular PP intervals and an isoelectric baseline. (Source: https://litfl.com/multifocal-atrial-tachycardia-mat-ecg-library/)

paroxysmal, persistent (>7 days), long-standing (≥1 year), or permanent persistent (≥1 year where rhythm control strategy is no longer attempted).[21]

ECG features include irregular atrial activity; absence of specific P-wave morphology; variable RR intervals; and absence of an isoelectric line. See **Fig. 12**.

The underlying pathophysiology of AF is an interplay between triggered activity and re-entry, requiring rapid triggered activity from an atrial ectopic focus (most often from

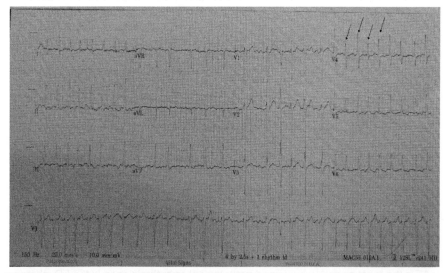

Fig. 12. AF with Rapid Ventricular Response: In this ECG, there is an irregularly irregular tachycardia at a rate of 116 bpm with narrow QRS complexes, variable RR intervals, and an absence of clear P-waves. Note the "QRS alternans" (*arrows*) that can occur in NCTs at rapid rates.

the muscle sleeve of the pulmonary vein) with sustained activity due to single or multiple reentrant circuits. Atrial remodeling (structural and electrical changes) results in variable refractoriness and conduction that can predispose to the development and maintenance of AF.[22]

Rapid and irregular atrial impulses fire at a rate of 400 to 700 bpm, most of which are not conducted through the AVN due to its refractoriness, leading to irregular ventricular beats at rates of 100 to 200 bpm or slower (<100 bpm) in untreated patients with AVN disease. Rates of over 200 to 220 bpm may occur if the refractory period of the AVN is shortened (eg, increased catecholamines) or in the presence of an AP conducting the impulses.

One-third of patients in AF are asymptomatic. Those coming to the ED with symptoms can have a presentation and complaints similar to those with other tachydysrhythmias, such as palpitations, breathlessness, dizziness, chest discomfort, or they can present with thromboembolic complications of AF, such as stroke, transient ischemic attack, or acute bowel or limb ischemia.[23]

AF occurs in those with structural cardiac causes, such as heart disease (eg, coronary, hypertensive, congenital, valvular, infiltrative), cardiomyopathy, heart failure, sick sinus syndrome, and preexcitation syndrome, which predispose patients to primary disease and chronicity. It is important to realize that AF is often the result of noncardiac pathophysiologic mechanisms (ie, sepsis, pulmonary embolism, electrolyte and acid–base disturbances, drugs, thyrotoxicosis, and pheochromocytoma) that can predispose patients to AF or AFL, or worsen AF episodes in patients with known AF.[24]

Special considerations in the treatment of atrial fibrillation and atrial flutter

Most cases of AF or AFL with a rapid ventricular response present with symptoms related to the arrhythmia. The first step is assessing the need for cardioversion (electrical or chemical), ventricular rate slowing therapy, and the need for antithrombotic agents.

Management decisions in AF/AFL should take into consideration the factors established in the 2021 CAEP best practice checklist for AF/AFL:

Determining if the AF/AFL is a primary condition or secondary to an underlying disease. Treatment of AF or AFL resulting from an underlying noncardiac etiology should focus on treating the underlying cause. Premature focus on rate or rhythm control in these patients (eg, giving a rate control agent to someone with underlying sepsis or pulmonary embolism) can result in deleterious consequences and hemodynamic collapse. Once AF/AFL is determined to be a primary issue, the next step is to *assess for hemodynamic instability*. Hypotension or signs of shock, active cardiac ischemia, or acute pulmonary edema should prompt initiation of rapid rhythm control using synchronized electrical cardioversion. In stable patients with no underlying etiologies and no signs of hemodynamic instability, treatment can occur with either rate or rhythm control. Both approaches are considered class 1, level B recommendations by the American Heart Association and the American College of Cardiology.[21] The RACE-7 study, published in 2019, shows no difference in ED discharge rates, return visits, or cardiovascular complications in those receiving cardioversion versus rate control in the ED.[25] *Rhythm control* can be achieved by electrical or chemical cardioversion. However, because of the risk of thromboembolic events after cardioversion, rhythm control should only be considered in (1) those with a clear onset of less than 48 hours, with some studies suggesting less than 12 hours[26,27] and (2) those who have been properly anticoagulated for more than 3 weeks. Chemical cardioversion can be achieved using a variety of agents, for example, procainamide, amiodarone, flecainide, dofetilide, propafenone, and IV ibutilide.[28,29]

In stable patients, *rate control* is more appropriate than rhythm control in those with an unknown, or prolonged, duration of AF/AFL, elderly patients (>65 years of age), those with valvular disease, or a high risk of stroke if cardioverted. Rate control can be achieved by administering beta-blockers or non-dihydropyridine CCB. Digoxin is less preferred in the ED setting. A heart rate goal of 110 bpm is a reasonable goal for patients with normal ejection fraction.[21,30]

Future stroke is a concern in patients with AF/AFL and(AC) may be required. Embolic risk in patients with AF is estimated using the CHA2DS2-VASc or the CHADS65 risk models. AC is required in all patients with a CHA2DS2-VASc score of greater than 1, a positive CHADS65, with a mechanical valve, or with moderate-to-severe mitral stenosis. The initiation of AC must be weighed against the risk of bleeding, using bleeding scores as an aid to that decision.

SUMMARY

NCTs are encountered regularly in the ED. It is incumbent on the emergency physician to perform a proper clinical assessment and carefully scrutinize the ECG to identify if the NCT at hand is a result, or cause, of the patient's condition. The ability to narrow the differential diagnosis of NCT by rhythm regularity can play an important role in proper identification of the arrhythmia and guide appropriate and timely management; from performing vagal maneuvers, administering effective medications, to delivering synchronized electrical cardioversion or focusing on treating the underlying cause, and, most importantly, avoiding unnecessary iatrogenic harm or discomfort.

CLINICS CARE POINTS

- The differential diagnosis for the most commonly encountered regular narrow complex tachycardia (NCT) in the emergency department includes:
  - Sinus tachycardia
  - Atrial flutter (AFL) with fixed 2:1 or 3:1 conduction
  - Supraventricular tachycardia (ie, atrioventricular nodal re-entrant tachycardia, orthodromic atrioventricular reciprocating tachycardia)
- The differential diagnosis for commonly encountered irregular NCTs includes
  - Atrial fibrillation (AF)
  - AFL with variable conduction
  - Multifocal atrial tachycardia
- Care should be taken to properly assess if the NCT is a result, or cause, of the patient's condition, as management options and goals greatly differ between the two.
- Understanding the pathophysiology behind NCTs can guide appropriate treatment options.
- Treatment of AF/AFL depends on multiple factors, including clinical stability, arrhythmia duration, and anticoagulation status.

DISCLOSURE

The authors have nothing to disclose.

REFERENCES

1. Probst MA, Mower WR, Kanzaria HK, et al. Analysis of emergency department visits for palpitations (from the National Hospital Ambulatory Medical Care Survey). Am J Cardiol 2014;113(10):1685–90.

2. Weber BE, Kapoor WN. Evaluation and outcomes of patients with palpitations. Am J Med 1996;100(2):138–48.
3. Orejarena LA, Vidaillet H, Destefano F, et al. Paroxysmal supraventricular tachycardia in the general population. J Am Coll Cardiol 1998;31(1):150–7.
4. Ganz LI, Friedman PL. Supraventricular tachycardia. N Engl J Med 1995;332(3): 162–73.
5. Ferguson JD, DiMarco JP. Contemporary management of paroxysmal supraventricular tachycardia. Circulation 2003;107(8):1096–9.
6. Brugada J, Katritsis DG, Arbelo E, et al. 2019 ESC Guidelines for the management of patients with supraventricular tachycardiaThe Task Force for the management of patients with supraventricular tachycardia of the European Society of Cardiology (ESC). Eur Heart J 2020;41(5):655–720.
7. Stahmer SA, Cowan R. Tachydysrhythmias. Emerg Med Clin North Am 2006; 24(1):11–40.
8. Cosío FG. Atrial flutter, typical and atypical: a review. Arrhythmia Electrophysiol Rev 2017;6(2):55.
9. Porter MJ, Morton JB, Denman R, et al. Influence of age and gender on the mechanism of supraventricular tachycardia. Hear Rhythm 2004;1(4):393–6.
10. Wood KA, Drew BJ, Scheinman MM. Frequency of disabling symptoms in supraventricular tachycardia. Am J Cardiol 1997;79(2):145–9.
11. González-Torrecilla E, Almendral J, Arenal A, et al. Combined evaluation of bedside clinical variables and the electrocardiogram for the differential diagnosis of paroxysmal atrioventricular reciprocating tachycardias in patients without preexcitation. J Am Coll Cardiol 2009;53(25):2353–8.
12. Kalusche D, Ott P, Arentz T, et al. AV nodal re-entry tachycardia in elderly patients. Coron Artery Dis 1998;9(6):359–64.
13. Page RL, Joglar JA, Caldwell MA, et al. 2015 ACC/AHA/HRS guideline for the management of adult patients with supraventricular tachycardia: a report of the american college of cardiology/american heart association task force on clinical practice guidelines and the heart rhythm society 2016;133. https://doi.org/10.1161/CIR.0000000000000311.
14. Smith G, Morgans A, Boyle M. Use of the Valsalva manoeuvre in the prehospital setting: a review of the literature. Emerg Med J 2009;26(1):8–10.
15. Taylor DMD, Wong LF. Incorrect instruction in the use of the Valsalva manoeuvre for paroxysmal supra-ventricular tachycardia is common. Emerg Med Australas 2004;16(4):284–7.
16. Appelboam A, Reuben A, Mann C, et al. Postural modification to the standard Valsalva manoeuvre for emergency treatment of supraventricular tachycardias (REVERT): a randomised controlled trial. Lancet 2015;386(10005):1747–53.
17. Corbacıoglu ŞK, Akıncı E, Çevik Y, et al. Comparing the success rates of standard and modified Valsalva maneuvers to terminate PSVT: A randomized controlled trial. Am J Emerg Med 2017;35(11):1662–5.
18. Brubaker S, Long B, Koyfman A. Alternative treatment options for atrioventricular-nodal-reentry tachycardia: an emergency medicine review. J Emerg Med 2018; 54(2):198–206.
19. Alabed S, Providência R, Chico TJA. Cochrane corner: adenosine versus intravenous calcium channel antagonists for supraventricular tachycardia. Heart 2018; 104(24):1993–4.
20. Goudis CA, Konstantinidis AK, Ntalas IV, et al. Electrocardiographic abnormalities and cardiac arrhythmias in chronic obstructive pulmonary disease. Int J Cardiol 2015;199:264–73.

21. January CT, Wann LS, Calkins H, et al. 2019 AHA/ACC/HRS focused update of the 2014 AHA/ACC/HRS guideline for the management of patients with atrial fibrillation: a report of the american college of cardiology/american heart association task force on clinical practice guidelines and the Heart R. Circulation 2019; 140(2):e125–51.

22. Thijssen VL, Ausma J, Liu GS, et al. Structural changes of atrial myocardium during chronic atrial fibrillation. Cardiovasc Pathol 2000;9(1):17–28.

23. Gibbs H, Freedman B, Rosenqvist M, et al. Clinical Outcomes in Asymptomatic and Symptomatic Atrial Fibrillation Presentations in GARFIELD-AF: Implications for AF Screening. Am J Med 2021;134(7):893–901.e11.

24. Fuster V, Rydén LE, Cannom DS, et al. ACC/AHA/ESC 2006 guidelines for the management of patients with atrial fibrillation: A report of the American College of Cardiology/American Heart Association Task Force on practice guidelines and the European Society of Cardiology Committee for practice. Circulation 2006;114(7):e257–354.

25. Pluymaekers NAHA, Dudink EAMP, Luermans JGLM, et al. Early or delayed cardioversion in recent-onset atrial fibrillation. N Engl J Med 2019;380(16):1499–508.

26. Andrade JG, Verma A, Mitchell LB, et al. 2018 Focused update of the canadian cardiovascular society guidelines for the management of atrial fibrillation. Can J Cardiol 2018;34(11):1371–92.

27. Airaksinen KEJ, Grönberg T, Nuotio I, et al. Thromboembolic complications after cardioversion of acute atrial fibrillation. J Am Coll Cardiol 2013;62(13):1187–92.

28. Oral H, Souza JJ, Michaud GF, et al. Facilitating transthoracic cardioversion of atrial fibrillation with ibutilide pretreatment. N Engl J Med 1999;340(24):1849–54.

29. Fibrillation AEP on A. ACEP AFIB evidence-driven tool to guide the selection and management of emergency department patients with atrial fibrillation and atrial flutter. Available at: https://www.acep.org/patient-care/afib/. Accessed December 23, 2021.

30. Hindricks G, Potpara T, Dagres N, et al. 2020 ESC Guidelines for the diagnosis and management of atrial fibrillation developed in collaboration with the European Association for Cardio-Thoracic Surgery (EACTS). Eur Heart J 2021; 42(5):373–498.

Wide Complex Tachycardias

Leen Alblaihed, MBBS, MHA[a],*, Tareq Al-Salamah, MBBS, MPH[a,b]

KEYWORDS

- Wide complex tachycardia • Ventricular tachycardia • Tachydysrhythmia
- Tachycardia

KEY POINTS

- Causes of wide complex tachycardia (WCT) range from benign (eg, sinus tachycardia with left bundle branch block) to malignant (eg, ventricular tachycardia [VT]).
- The most critical task in managing WCT is determining whether the tachyarrhythmia has a ventricular or supraventricular origin in order to initiate appropriate treatment. This can be achieved by obtaining a good clinical history and scrutinizing the 12-lead electrocardiogram (ECG).
- WCT with a uniform morphology should be presumed to be VT and managed as such. If gone untreated, it can lead to decompensation and death.
- Knowing the ECG findings of VT can help in diagnosis; however, there exists types of narrow complex VT that make diagnosis challenging in the emergency department.

INTRODUCTION

Wide refers to a QRS complex duration of $\geq$0.12 seconds (120 milliseconds), or 3 small boxes on the electrocardiographic (ECG) paper, and *tachycardia* is defined as greater than 100 beats/min (bpm). Wide complex tachycardia (WCT) is commonly seen on the 12-lead ECG recordings of patients in the emergency department (ED). A widened QRS duration essentially means that ventricular depolarization (activation) is abnormally slow. In WCT, the impulse could originate from the atria (supraventricular), but is abnormally propagated through the ventricles, or originate from the ventricles (outside of the conduction system) with direct muscle activation. To be able to differentiate between the causes of WCT, it is important to understand the following: (1) Why the QRS complex is wide, and (2) Why there is tachycardia.

[a] Department of Emergency Medicine, University of Maryland School of Medicine, Baltimore, MD, USA; [b] Department of Emergency Medicine, King Saud University, PO Box 7805, Riyadh 11472, Saudi Arabia
* Corresponding author. 110 South Paca Street, Sixth Floor, Suite 200, Baltimore, MD 21201.
E-mail address: lalblaihed@som.umaryland.edu
Twitter: @LeenAlblaihed (L.A.); @SalamahTareq (T.A.-S.)

Emerg Med Clin N Am 40 (2022) 733–753
https://doi.org/10.1016/j.emc.2022.06.010
0733-8627/22/© 2022 Elsevier Inc. All rights reserved.

Causes of Wide QRS Complexes

Abnormalities in conduction of atrial impulses to the ventricles

Normally, electrical impulses (or depolarizing waves) that start in the atria and pass through the atrioventricular node (AVN) are propagated rapidly and near simultaneously to the ventricles via the His-Purkinje network. The fast-conducting bundle of His divides into the right and left bundle branches (RBB and LBB). The LBB further divides into the anterior and posterior fascicles. These bundles progressively divide to form an intricate Purkinje network covering most of the endocardial surface of the ventricles.[1,2]

Abnormalities related to the conduction system can occur either owing to a dysfunction of the His-Purkinje network or to the presence of an abnormal (accessory) pathway where an impulse can be directly conducted to the ventricular myocardial cells initiating a slower depolarization.

Dysfunctional His-Purkinje system. Parts (branches) of the fast conducting His-Purkinje ventricular network may lose the ability to rapidly propagate the depolarization wave. Damage to the physical structure of the network fibers (eg, fibrosis, post-ischemic scarring) or physiologic inhibition of its function (eg, electrolyte abnormalities, membrane receptor blockage) will result in a slower depolarization wave and a wide QRS complex. This abnormal conduction through the ventricles is also termed "aberrancy."[3]

a. Preexisting bundle branch block (BBB): There is intrinsic impairment (delay or blockage) of conduction through the bundle branches or Purkinje system. When a supraventricular tachycardia (SVT) occurs in a patient with a baseline BBB, the QRS complex should have a typical BBB (right or left) morphology. When available, reviewing prior ECGs should demonstrate similar QRS morphology (**Fig. 1**).

b. Rate-related aberrancy (functional aberrancy): The basic premise of this phenomenon is the premature arrival of an impulse before the conduction has recovered from its refractory state from the previous beat.[3] Refractoriness is influenced by rate and preceding cycle length. The refractory duration of the proximal right bundle is longer than that of the left bundle.[4] In atrial tachycardias (eg, SVT or atrial

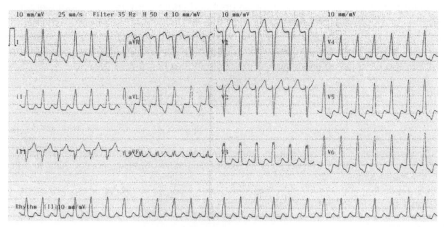

Fig. 1. SVT with aberrant conduction. This ECG shows a WCT owing to a fixed LBBB, and the tachycardia is due to AVNRT. Note, there is no Q wave in V6 (typical of LBBB). Prior ECG of the patient (not included) also reveals the LBBB. (Image source litfl.com.)

fibrillation [AF]) when 1 impulse is shortly followed by another impulse, it may find the RBB in a refractory period (functionally blocked) resulting in a wide QRS complex with right bundle branch block (RBBB) morphology. This is the basis behind the Ashmann phenomenon seen in AF[5] (**Fig. 2**). The refractory period depends on the heart rate (HR) (ie, the RR interval). When the HR is fast, the RR interval is short. Short cardiac cycles have shorter refractory periods. Oppositely, when the HR is slow, there is a long RR interval, and a longer refractory period. When a long RR interval is followed by an early impulse (short RR), it will encounter refractory fibers (typically the RBB fibers), resulting in a wide QRS complex. This can sometimes lead to a run of aberrantly conducted beats mistaken for VT.[6]

c. Dysfunction or delay of the intraventricular conduction system can also occur owing to various factors.[7]

- Electrolyte abnormalities (eg, hyperkalemia), metabolic derangements, toxidromes (eg, sodium channel toxicity, TCA overdose), medications (eg, AV nodal blockers, antiarrhythmics), and drugs can alter cardiomyocyte action potentials that may lead to slowing down or blocking impulse conduction, resulting in a myriad of ECG changes, including WCT[7,8] (**Fig. 3**).

- Myocardial infarction (MI) can cause scarring and damage to the conduction system, resulting in BBB or interventricular delays widening the QRS complex. At a cellular level, MI can cause ionic imbalances and loss of gap junction function that result in slower conduction, and ST elevations that can mimic wide complex rhythms[7,9] (**Fig. 4**).

Accessory pathway. An accessory pathway (AP) is an electrically conducting pathway, existing outside the normal conducting system, that connects the atria to the ventricles bypassing the AVN.[10] The term "preexcitation" refers to the ventricles being depolarized earlier via the AP than normal conduction via the AVN.[10,11] Conduction to the ventricles can occur entirely via the AP (maximal preexcitation), entirely via the AVN (no preexcitation), or via both pathways, creating fusion complexes that

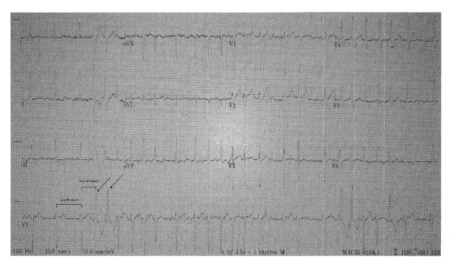

Fig. 2. AF with RVR and Ashmann' phenomenon. In this ECG, the patient is in AF with RVR with 2 episodes of 2 consecutive wide QRS beats (*arrows*) that occurred after a short RR interval that followed a long RR interval, hallmark of Ashmann phenomenon.

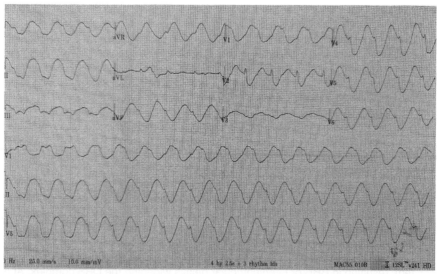

Fig. 3. Hyperkalemia. Regular tachycardia with a rightward axis, no clear P waves, and very wide QRS complexes (>160milliseconds) with a "sine wave" appearance concerning for hyperkalemia.

can show varying degrees of preexcitation.[12] In preexcitation, impulses that travel anterogradely down the AP activate the ventricles outside the normal fast conducting system, resulting in a widened QRS complex.[10] Wolf-Parkinson-White syndrome (WPW) is the most common preexcitation syndrome[13] (**Figs. 5** and **6**).

Impulses generated in the ventricles
The most critical task in managing WCT is determining whether the tachyarrhythmia has a ventricular or supraventricular origin in order to initiate appropriate treatment.[14]

- A wide QRS complex can also be caused by an impulse originating in the ventricular tissues. The depolarization wave propagates and spreads from the site of

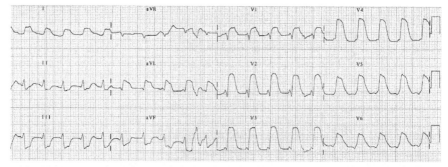

Fig. 4. Tombstone ST segment elevation MI. In this ECG, massive ST elevation with "tombstone" morphology is present throughout the precordial (V1-6) and high lateral leads (I, aVL) This pattern is seen in proximal left anterior descending artery occlusion and indicates a large territory infarction with a poor LV ejection fraction and high likelihood of cardiogenic shock and death. (Image source: litfl.com.)

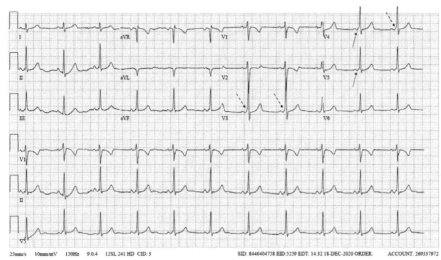

Fig. 5. WPW. In this ECG, the patient is in normal sinus rhythm at a rate of 65 bpm. The PR interval is short (<120 milliseconds) (*solid arrows*), and there is a slurring of the upstroke at the beginning of the QRS complex ("Delta wave") (*dashed arrows*) suggesting ventricular "pre-excitation" through an AP, as is the case with WPW.

origin, remote from the normal conduction system, using the much slower cardiomyocyte-to-cardiomyocyte conduction. In impulses generated outside of the conductive tissue, there will be a delayed "slurred" initial component of the QRS complex and a longer time to the peak of the R wave (ie, R-wave peak time) in comparison to those seen in impulses with aberrant conductions because of the initial partial conductions via the preserved His-Purkinje components.[15,16] However, once the ectopic ventricular impulse engages the conduction system and activates the remainder of the myocardium, the terminal components of the QRS will show a more rapid, sharper, deflection.[17] It is imperative to know what a typical left bundle branch block (LBBB) and RBBB QRS morphology look like in order to recognize the atypical QRS morphologies that are seen with VT.

- A wide QRS complex will also be seen with both right ventricle and biventricular pacing. Single-ventricle pacing typically originates from the right ventricular (RV) apex leading to a QRS morphology that mimics an LBBB except in leads V5-V6, which will almost always be negatively oriented in a paced rhythm.

Causes of Tachycardias with Wide QRS Complexes

WCT occurs owing to either (1) A nonventricular originating tachycardia (ie, SVT that is conducted abnormally to the ventricles), or (2) Ventricular originating tachycardia (VT).

Supraventricular tachycardia with abnormal ventricular conduction

The wide QRS complex in this type of tachycardia is a result of the impulse traversing the ventricles aberrantly through the normal conduction system or via an AP leading to preexcitation of ventricular myocardium. In these situations, ventricular myocardium does not dictate HR or rhythm; rather, they are dictated by the origin of the SVT, and the conductance capacity of the tissue carrying the electrical impulses to the ventricles. The ECG will show features of that respective tachycardia along with features

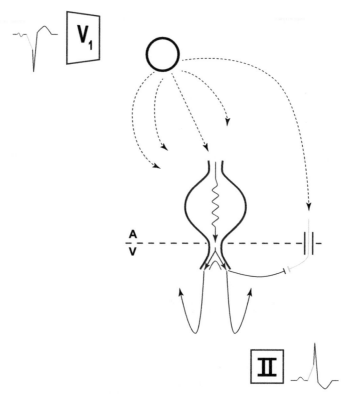

Fig. 6. Ventricular preexcitation. An atrioventricular AP allows conduction of electrical impulse from the atria (*dashed arrows*) to the ventricle directly, bypassing the AVN, leading to ventricular "preexcitation" (*gray arrow*), which is reflected on ECG as short PR with an up-slurring of the QRS complex "Delta-wave." (Figure courtesy of Dr. AbdulAziz AlKanhal)

of the respective cause of aberrant conduction. If the rhythm generated in the atria is regular (eg, atrioventricular reentrant tachycardia [AVRT], sinus tachycardia), the ECG will show a *regular* WCT, but if the supraventricular rhythm is irregular (eg, AF), this will result in an *irregular* WCT.

Below are examples of WCT with a supraventricular origin.

a. *Sinus tachycardia* with a fixed (eg, preexisting BBB) or rate-related BBB. The ECG will show positively oriented P waves in leads I, II, III; a consistent P-wave–QRS complex relationship for each beat; HR typically 100 to 160 bpm; QRS complex morphology consistent with a BBB[18] (**Fig. 7**).
b. *AF* is more common in elderly and those with structural heart disease. It can present with a rapid ventricular response (RVR), in which case the QRS complex can be wide owing to a fixed or rate-related BBB. The ECG will show absence of P waves, wide QRS complex with consistent morphology, and irregular RR interval.

When an *AP* is present (eg, WPW), the ECG will show extremely rapid ventricular rates (>240 bpm) and beat to beat QRS morphology changes (owing to fusion beats with different contributions from accessory and AVN conduction). Of note, there is similar concern in atrial flutter in the presence of an AP (**Fig. 8**).

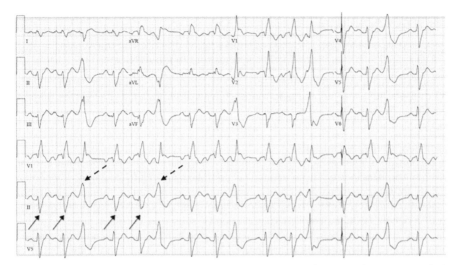

Fig. 7. Sinus tachycardia with RBBB and PVCs (trigeminy). In this ECG, there is a regularly irregular rhythm, and every third beat is a PVC (trigeminy). The rhythm is sinus (ie, P wave for every QRS, except the PVCs, upright in inferior leads and inverted in V1) at a rate around 100 bpm with wide QRS complexes. The sinus QRS complexes (*solid arrows*) meet criteria for RBBB. The premature ventricular contraction (PVC) (*dashed arrow*) follows every 2 sinus beats. Diagnosis: Sinus tachycardia with RBBB with ventricular trigeminy.

c. *Atrioventricular nodal reentrant tachycardia (AVNRT)*, can have a wide QRS because of a fixed or rate-related BBB. The ECG will show rapid rates (120–260 bpm, typically 170–180 bpm), wide QRS (120–140 milliseconds), and the absence of normal P waves (70% retrograde P waves).

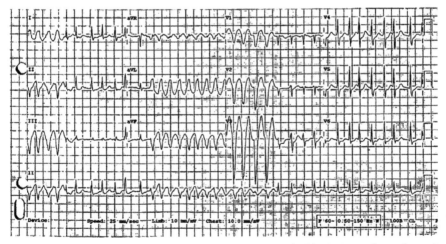

Fig. 8. AF with an AP. In this ECG, there is intermittent rapid wide QRS complex tachycardia of varying QRS morphologies suggestive of AF with intermittent conduction at a rate of 215 bpm with 1:1 conduction through an AP. AF in the context of an AP (eg, WPW) can be life-threatening if left untreated and can be deadly if mistreated with AV nodal blocking agents, which would lead to all atrial fibrillatory impulses going to the ventricles through the AP.

d. *Antidromic AVRT (eg, WPW)* can be a malignant rhythm owing to extreme ventricular rates reaching 180 to 260 bpm. The impulse goes down (anterograde) the AP, traverses the ventricles, and then conducts retrograde back up the AVN to the atria. This is an "antidromic" conduction with respect to the AVN.

The ECG will show rapid rates (180–260 bpm), regular rhythm, wide QRS (120–160 milliseconds) with unchanging morphologies, and absence of P waves (**Figs. 9** and **10**).

Ventricular Generated Impulses

Ventricular generated impulses encompass a large spectrum of abnormal cardiac rhythms from single premature ventricular complexes (PVC) to sustained monomorphic VT (MVT), polymorphic VT (PVT), and ventricular fibrillation. Their presentation ranges from asymptomatic to sudden cardiac death.[19] Most of these arrhythmias occur in patients with underlying structural heart disease (eg, cardiomyopathies); however, they still can occur in those without underlying cardiac disease (ie, idiopathic).[20] Impulses can be generated from any part of the intraventricular conduction system or ventricular myocardium.[21]

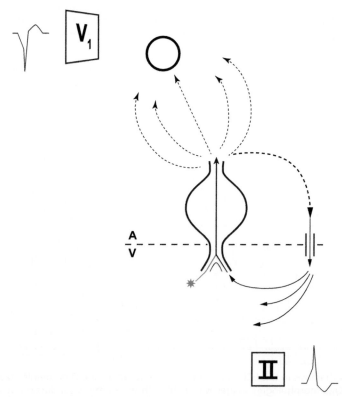

Fig. 9. Antidromic AVRT. A reentrant circuit develops where the electrical impulse travels from ventricles (*solid arrows*) through the AVN retrogradely spreading through the atria (*dashed arrows*) and then back to the ventricles anterogradely through an AP. Note QRS complexes are wide owing to ventricular depolarization through the AP. (Figure courtesy of Dr. AbdulAziz AlKanhal)

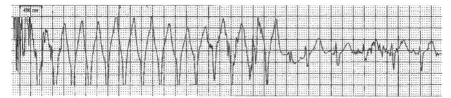

Fig. 10. Antidromic AVRT. There is an episode of a rapid regular tachycardia at a rate around 200 bpm with wide QRS complexes owing to ventricular "preexcitation" through an AP. Note the unchanging morphologies. P waves may be absent (buried) or retrograde. The differential diagnosis includes ventricular tachycardia, or any regular SVT with aberrant conduction.

VENTRICULAR TACHYCARDIA

Defined as a series of 3 or more consecutive wide complex beats with a rate greater than 120 bpm, VT usually ranges from 130 to 200 bpm, typically more than 170 bpm.[7,21] VT rates can be slower (130–160 bpm) in patients on amiodarone or with severe dilated cardiomyopathy.[7] A series of more than 3 wide complex beats at rates between 100 and 120 bpm is referred to as accelerated idioventricular rhythm and should not be confused with VT, as they are transient and occur after reperfusion after MI.[6,7] VT is termed sustained when there is hemodynamic instability, or it lasts for greater than 30 seconds.[22]

PATHOPHYSIOLOGY

The underlying mechanisms of VT, similar to other tachyarrhythmias, can be divided into 3 broad categories: reentrant, triggered activity, or abnormal automaticity.[23]

Reentry requires a trigger (eg, PVC) and a "loop" or 2 connected pathways (eg, scar or fibrosis from prior MI, surgery, cardiomyopathy) that differ in conduction speed and refractoriness to initiate and sustain the arrhythmia, respectively. Reentry is the underlying mechanism for most sustained VT in the presence of structural heart disease.[24,25] However, functional reentry (without anatomic scars) can also occur[19] (**Fig. 11**).

Triggered activity results from the premature activation of the cardiac cells by afterdepolarization. Simply, it is when a new depolarization occurs during or after the repolarization phase. They include early afterdepolarization (EAD) and delayed after depolarization (DAD) depending on the phase of cardiac action potential.

Automaticity, either enhanced or abnormal, may arise from a subordinate pacemaker in the His-Purkinje system or ventricular myocardium.[19]

TYPES OF VENTRICULAR TACHYCARDIA

VT can be divided by its morphology into monomorphic, polymorphic, pleomorphic, or bidirectional (**Table 1**). *MVT* arises from the same ventricular focus and has a uniform QRS morphology and a constant rate in any single lead[7] (**Fig. 12**). On ECG, MVT is frequently confused with other types of WCT, particularly SVT with aberrancy owing to their similar appearance. Distinguishing ECG features of both are mentioned in **Table 2**[17]; however, in any WCT that shows atypical features of a BBB morphology, VT should be suspected. MVT has been further classified into "classic VT" and "idiopathic VT." Idiopathic VT encompasses the following: (1) Right ventricular outflow tract (RVOT) VT, (2) Fascicular VT, and (3) Bundle branch reentrant tachycardia (**Table 3**. In

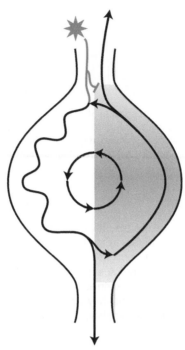

Fig. 11. The basics of reentrant loops (circuits). Any reentrant loop is usually made up of 2 pathways, 1 pathway with fast conduction but slow recovery (long refractory period), and the other with slower conduction and a faster recovery period. (Macro reentry = circuits are big enough to be mapped, eg, atrial flutter, AVRT. Micro reentry = circuit is too small to be mapped; AF, intra-atrial reentrant tachycardia). (Figure courtesy of Dr. AbdulAziz AlKanhal)

general, idiopathic VT frequently uses (or are near) the intrinsic conduction system; they have a steep initial portion of the QRS, and their QRS is generally narrower (<140milliseconds) than that of classic VT. It can be very difficult to distinguish them from SVT with aberrancy or classic VT (**Fig. 13**).

Table 1
Types of ventricular tachycardia by QRS morphology

Monomorphic	Pleomorphic	Polymorphic	Bidirectional
Single morphology QRS	More than 1 morphology for QRS, but morphology not continuously changing	Continuously changing QRS morphology; grouped into long QT and normal QT interval	Rare, beat-to-beat alternation of the QRS axis 180°; changes axis from left to right with each beat Associated with severe digoxin toxicity; also present in familial catecholaminergic polymorphic VT

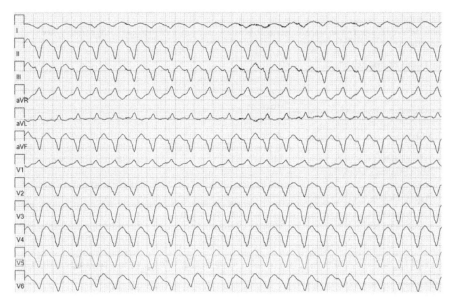

Fig. 12. MVT. In this ECG, there is a tachycardia at a rate of 147 bpm with 1 wide QRS complex (>120 milliseconds) with 1 morphology ("monomorphic"). A.

In contrast, *PVT* (**Table 4**) arises from more than 1 ventricular focus and has variable QRS morphologies and variable rate in any single lead.[7] PVT occurs in patients with underlying myocardial ischemia ion channel disorders (eg, long QT syndrome, Brugada syndrome), catecholaminergic PVT, and idiopathic ventricular fibrillation.[20] Torsades de pointes (twisting of points) is a subtype of PVT occurring in those with a prolonged QTc interval on their baseline ECG. It is characterized by a changing amplitude and polarity of the QRS complex whereby it is twisting around the isoelectric line (**Fig. 14**). The mechanism of torsades is through triggered activity whereby EAD occurs in the setting of an acquired or congenital prolongation of the QTc interval. The risk of torsades increases significantly when the QTc is greater than 500 mseconds. PVT with a normal QTc interval can look similar to torsades; however, it occurs in cardiac ischemia or infarction, and patients are usually unstable, requiring defibrillation.

MIMICS OF WIDE COMPLEX TACHYCARDIA

Some conditions exist that may present with a WCT that can be mistaken for VT owing to similarities on the 12-lead ECG. Examples include severe hyperkalemia, sodium channel blocker toxicity (eg, tricyclic antidepressant overdose), electrolyte and metabolic derangements, large ST-elevation MI (ie, tombstone elevations), postcardiac arrest rhythms, and artifact. Careful scrutiny of the ECG, clinical evaluation, and history will help differentiate these conditions from VT.

MANAGEMENT OF WIDE COMPLEX TACHYCARDIA IN THE EMERGENCY DEPARTMENT

WCT can present a diagnostic and therapeutic challenge to the emergency physician, especially with difficulty accessing older ECGs for comparison. The differential for WCT is wide and includes VT, SVT with aberrant conduction, preexcitation

Table 2
The differences between ventricular tachycardia and supraventricular tachycardia with aberrancy

SVT with Aberrancy	VT	
	Usually in those with prior history of MI, heart disease	
Baseline sinus ECG may show • WPW • QRS complex abnormalities related to medication or hyperkalemia	Baseline sinus ECG may show • Q waves indicative of old MI • Prolonged QT interval • Brugada syndrome	Preexisting BBB can be a helpful indicator for SVT with aberrancy; however, BBB occurs in chronic heart disease, therefore increased chance of VT
AV dissociation can rarely occur in AVNRT	AV dissociation occurs in 50% of VT. Its absence does not exclude VT	In VT without retrograde conduction to the atria, sinus rhythm continues independently from the ventricular activity, resulting in AVD
	Capture beats	An ideally timed supraventricular beat will be conducted down the normal pathway resulting in ventricular depolarization and a QRS complex that resembles patient's baseline QRS
	Fusion beats	A supraventricular depolarization wave conducted down the AVN, collides and "fuses" with a ventricular depolarization wave originating in the ventricle. They form a hybrid QRS complex with different morphology than the other MVT beats

https://doi.org/10.1161/JAHA.120.016598.

syndromes, hyperkalemia, and other metabolic and toxic drug effects. The treatment of the listed conditions differs vastly, and worse, specific treatments for some can be detrimental in others. There have been many publications and guidelines describing algorithms to help differentiate these rhythms; however, they performed poorly at the bedside and can lead to mismanagement and harm.[7,26]

REGULAR WIDE COMPLEX TACHYCARDIA

The majority (80%) of regular WCT are due to VT, especially if they have underlying structural heart disease, a history of MI, or heart failure.[7,27,28] The different algorithms to differentiate WCT are too complex, difficult to recall, and inaccurate in the clinical setting.[29] Therefore, in the ED, any regular WCT should be assumed VT until proven otherwise. Some ECG findings that strengthen the probability of VT are as follows:

Table 3
Types of monomorphic ventricular tachycardia

	Classic	Idiopathic		Bundle Branch Reentrant VT
		RVOT VT "Focal"	Fascicular VT	
	Most common cause of RWCT			
Location/origin	Originates in myocardium (outside conduction system)	Originating in RVOT, then accesses nearby conduction system	Originating in or near the intrinsic conduction system: • Posterior fascicle (most common 90%–95%) • Anterior fascicle (5%–10%) • Upper septal fascicle (rare)	Reentry circuit involving both bundle branches. Anterograde over RBB and retrograde over LBB
Mechanism		Triggered activity	Reentrant	Reentrant
Occurs in	Advanced age, CV disease, structural heart disease, ischemia	Younger age, associated with arrhythmogenic right ventricular dysplasia	Younger, no structural heart disease	Younger, with underlying structural heart disease
Prognosis	Has a worse prognosis and hemodynamic compromise	Better prognosis and less hemodynamic compromise	Better prognosis and less hemodynamic compromise	Due to extreme fast rates can cause, syncope or SCD

(continued on next page)

Table 3
(continued)

	Classic	Idiopathic		Bundle Branch Reentrant VT
		RVOT VT "Focal"	Fascicular VT	
Basic ECG features		PVCs, precordial LBBB pattern with inferior frontal plane axis	Precordial RBBB pattern with • LAFB (left axis) in posterior fascicle VT • LPFB (right axis) in anterior fascicular block	The QRS morphology is typical of a BBB (usually LBBB) and may look identical to the patient's sinus ECG. In sinus rhythm, most patients with BBRVT have a prolonged QRS (LBBB or nonspecific conduction delay), which makes it difficult to distinguish from WCT due to SVT with aberrancy
QRS	The first portion of QRS is conducted wide, and the QRS duration is usually >140 ms	Initial portion of QRS is rapid, steep, and organized Narrower (<140 ms)	Initial portion of QRS is rapid, steep, and organized Narrower (<140 ms)	Initial portion of QRS is rapid, steep, and organized Narrower (<140 ms)
LV function on ultrasound	Poor	Good	Good	Good
Treatment		Responsive to adenosine	Posterior fascicle responds to verapamil, anterior fascicle, no specific treatment	No specific pharmacologic treatment

Table 4
Types of ventricular tachycardia based on morphology

	MVT	PVT	
		TdP	Other PVT
QRS morphology	Uniform	2 or more different morphologies	2 or more different morphologies
Rate	Constant	Changing	Changing
ECG features	AV dissociation Fusion complexes Capture beats	Prolonged QTc	
Axis	Constant	Shifting in TdP	Constant
Mechanism	Structural abnormalities of the heart, reentry		Triggered (EAD, DAD) Automaticity
			Abnormal repolarization: in ACS, electrolyte abnormalities, medication toxicity Congenital

1) Inconsistent P-QRS relationship (AV dissociation); this was found in approximately 50% of cases of VT[28] (**Fig. 15** (2) QRS concordance in the chest leads (ie, all chest leads QRS complexes are in the same direction) with a negative concordance being more concerning for VT; (3) The presence of fusion beats, which are hybrid beats owing to ventricular activation from a conducted atrial impulse fused with a beat originating in the ventricle.

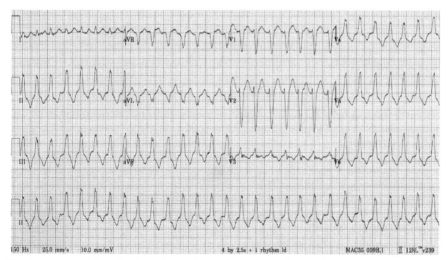

Fig. 13. RVOT VT. Regular broad complex tachycardia with LBBB-like morphology with RS complex in V1 and R complex in V6. Precordial transition at V3 inferior axis (+90°).

A

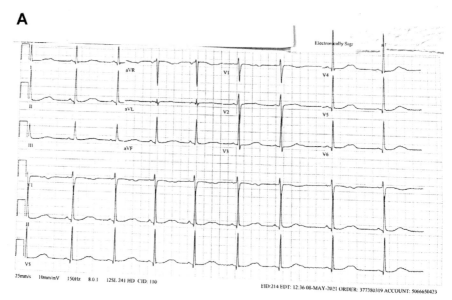

B

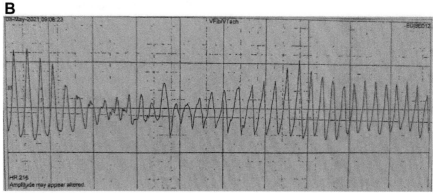

Fig. 14. (*A*) Prolonged QT. Sinus bradycardia with a prolonged QT interval. (*B*) Torsades de pointes: same patient, now in a WCT with more than 1 QRS morphology ("polymorphic") with varying amplitudes, and axes that appear to be twisting around a point ("torsades de pointes").

When managing regular WCT, it is best to treat it as VT. Unstable patients should undergo direct electric synchronized cardioversion. In stable patients with regular WCT, cardioversion is a reasonable first-line treatment especially in very fast HRs or evidence of left ventricular systolic dysfunction on bedside echocardiography. The success rate for electrical cardioversion for stable VT is 95% higher than the success rate of pharmacologic cardioversion.[30]

In clinically stable patients, another option is pharmacologic cardioversion. IV Procainamide is more effective and safer (with fewer side effects) than IV amiodarone for acute conversion of VT.[31]

In cases whereby SVT is strongly suspected, IV adenosine can be used for conversion. If the WCT is not terminated, then VT should be considered as probable. However, because a small percentage of VT can also be converted with adenosine,

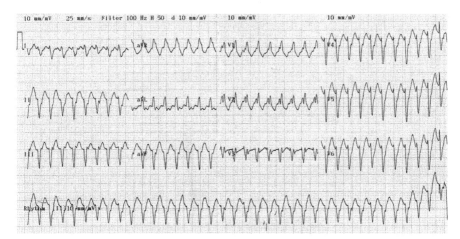

Fig. 15. MVT. The ECG shows a WCT (HR > 100, QRS > 120), and the appearance in V1 is more suggestive of SVT with aberrancy, given that the complexes are not that broad (<160 milliseconds) and the right rabbit ear is taller than the left. However, on closer inspection, there are signs of AV dissociation, with superimposed P waves visible in V1. Also, the presence of a northwest axis. Comparing to baseline ECG (not included), the patient had a completely different QRS axis and morphology on his baseline ECG. (Image source: litfl.com.)

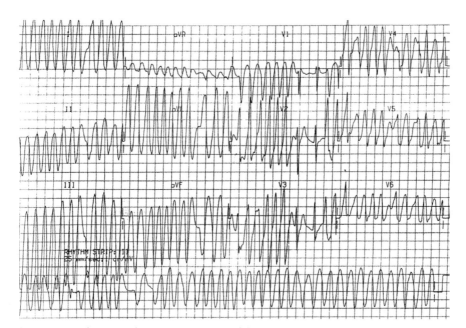

Fig. 16. AF with WPW. The ECG is a very rapid (up to 300 bpm in places), irregular broad-complex tachycardia with varying QRS morphologies. There are 2 narrow complexes (in V1-3) where the atrial impulses are presumably conducted via the AVN instead of via the AP. This rhythm is difficult to differentiate from PVT; however, it does not demonstrate the twisting morphology characteristic of torsades de pointes.

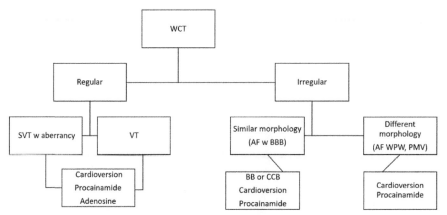

Fig. 17. Algorithm summarizing treatment of WCT in stable patients. Regular WCT should be managed as VT. They can be treated by cardioversion or procainamide. It is safe to use adenosine to diagnose or treat regular WCT. Irregular WCT of similar morphology are due to impulses using the same pathway (ANV) to reach the ventricle; these can be managed with BB or CCB, cardioversion, or procainamide. Irregular WCT is best treated with cardioversion or procainamide. BB, beta-blockers; CCB, calcium channel blockers.

adenosine cannot completely exclude VT as a diagnosis. The use of adenosine in WCT has been shown to be safe in regular WCT.[32]

Littmann and colleagues[28] described a few pitfalls and mistakes that need to be avoided when evaluating patients that present with a WCT on an ECG: (1) Automatically adopting another clinician's false diagnosis (anchoring bias), (2) Thinking the patient is "too well" for VT. Patients with VT can be clinically stable on presentation; they frequently become unstable as a result of a missed diagnosis and inappropriate treatment; (3) The "P-wave trap" occurs when a clinician focuses too much on a possible 1:1 P-QRS relationship thereby dismissing VT as a diagnosis, when in reality some VT will have a 1:1 retrograde conduction. In addition, part of the ST-T segment can be mistaken for a P wave; (4) Focusing on the QRS morphology resembling a BBB when the patient has other more concerning findings of VT, like AV dissociation.

IRREGULAR WIDE COMPLEX TACHYCARDIA

Sustained irregular WCT is almost never VT. The most likely diagnosis is atrial fibrillation with an abnormal conduction to the ventricles (ie, BBB, or AP). AF with a BBB is more likely when the QRS morphology is consistent. In AF with preexcitation (eg, WPW), the HR will be greater than 180 bpm, and the QRS morphology will vary (see **Fig. 8**).

Treatment of AF with a BBB is similar to treating narrow-complex AF (ie, rate or rhythm control). In cases of AF with an AP (**Fig. 16**), it is critical to avoid using AVN blocking agents. Medications like adenosine, calcium channel blockers, beta-blockers, digoxin, or amiodarone can be fatal owing to blocking AVN conduction, sending all the AF impulses down the rapidly conducting AP to the ventricles, leading to ventricular rates that approach or exceed 300 bpm.[33] Electric cardioversion is a reasonable initial treatment option. If pharmacologic agents are used, IV procainamide is the agent of choice, as it preferentially suppresses the AP (**Fig. 17**).

SUMMARY

WCTs are frequently encountered in the ED. Causes of WCT are broad and range from benign to life-threatening (eg, atrial fibrillation with WPW, or ventricular tachycardia). It is imperative that the emergency physician is familiar with the clinical presentation, underlying causes, and ECG features of the different causes of WCT. However, in a busy clinical setting, simplifying the approach to treatment by categorizing WCT into regular versus irregular might be the safest and easiest method. Regular WCT should always be presumed to be VT unless proven otherwise. Irregular WCT are rarely ventricular in origin.

CLINICS CARE POINTS

- A regular wide complex tachycardia should be presumed to be ventricular tachycardia and treated as such.
- Patients with ventricular tachycardia can be clinically stable initially but can decompensate quickly, so it is reasonable to prepare for electrical cardioversion even if pharmacologic therapy is initiated.
- Electrocardiographic features of benign and malignant causes of wide complex tachycardia can be confusing. Looking at prior electrocardiograms and knowing the typical left bundle branch block and right bundle branch block features can help identify ventricular tachycardia.

DISCLOSURE

The Authors have nothing to disclose.

REFERENCES

1. Syed FF, Hai JJ, Lachman N, et al. The infrahisian conduction system and endocavitary cardiac structures: relevance for the invasive electrophysiologist. J Interv Card Electrophysiol 2014;39(1):45–56.
2. Desplantez T, Dupont E, Severs NJ, et al. Gap Junction Channels and Cardiac Impulse Propagation. J Membr Biol 2007;218(1–3):13–28.
3. Pollack ML, Chan TC, Brady WJ. Electrocardiographic manifestations: aberrant ventricular conduction. J Emerg Med 2000;19(4):363–7.
4. Bailey JC, Lathrop DA, Pippenger DL. Differences between proximal left and right bundle branch block action potential durations and refractoriness in the dog heart. Circ Res 1977;40(5):464–8.
5. Singla V, Singh B, Singh Y, et al. Ashman phenomenon: a physiological aberration. Case Rep 2013;2013(may24 1). bcr2013009660.
6. Stahmer SA, Cowan R. Tachydysrhythmias Emerg Med Clin North Am 2006;24(1): 11–40.
7. Brady WJ, Mattu A, Tabas J, et al. The differential diagnosis of wide QRS complex tachycardia. Am J Emerg Med 2017;35(10):1525–9.
8. Parham WA, Mehdirad AA, Biermann KM, et al. Hyperkalemia revisited. Tex Hear Inst J 2006;33(1):40–7. Available at: http://www.ncbi.nlm.nih.gov/pubmed/16572868.
9. Janse MWAL. Electrophysiological mechanisms of ventricular arrhythmias resulting from myocardial ischemia and infarction. Physiol Rev 1989;69(4):1049–169.

10. Olgin JE, Zipes DP. Supraventricular Arrhythmias. In: Bonow R, Mann D, Tomaselli G, et al, editors. Braunwald's heart disease: a textbook of cardiovascular medicine. 11th edition. Elsevier Inc.; 2019. p. 706–29.

11. Murgatroyd F. Handbook of cardiac electrophysiology: a practical guide to invasive EP studies and catheter ablation. ReMEDICA Pub; 2002.

12. Olshansky B, Chung MK, Pogwizd SM, et al. Ventricular tachyarrhythmias. In: Olshansky B, Chung MK, Pogwizd SM, et al, editors. Arrhythmia essentials. 2nd edition. Elsevier; 2017. p. 219–77.

13. Wallace A. Cardiovascular disease. In: Pardo MC, Miller RD, editors. Basics of anesthesia. 7th edition. Elsevier Inc; 2018. p. 415–49.

14. Brady WJ, Skiles J. Wide QRS complex tachycardia: ECG differential diagnosis. Am J Emerg Med 1999;17(4):376–81.

15. Brugada P, Brugada J, Mont L, et al. A new approach to the differential diagnosis of a regular tachycardia with a wide QRS complex. Circulation 1991;83(5): 1649–59.

16. Pava LF, Perafán P, Badiel M, et al. R-wave peak time at DII: A new criterion for differentiating between wide complex QRS tachycardias. Hear Rhythm 2010;7(7): 922–6.

17. Kashou AH, Noseworthy PA, DeSimone CV, et al. Wide Complex Tachycardia Differentiation: A Reappraisal of the State-of-the-Art. J Am Heart Assoc 2020;9(11). https://doi.org/10.1161/JAHA.120.016598.

18. Smith S. Left bundle branch block. In: Smith S, Zvosec D, SW S, et al, editors. The ECG in acute MI: an evidence-based manual of reperfusion therapy. Lippincott Williams & Wilkins; 2002.

19. Al-Khatib SM, Stevenson WG, Ackerman MJ, et al. 2017 AHA/ACC/HRS Guideline for Management of Patients With Ventricular Arrhythmias and the Prevention of Sudden Cardiac Death. Circulation 2018;138(13). https://doi.org/10.1161/CIR. 0000000000000549.

20. Roberts-Thomson KC, Lau DH, Sanders P. The diagnosis and management of ventricular arrhythmias. Nat Rev Cardiol 2011;8(6):311–21.

21. Hudson KB, Brady WJ, Chan TC, et al. Electrocardiographic manifestations: ventricular tachycardia. J Emerg Med 2003;25(3):303–14.

22. Pires LA, Lehmann MH, Buxton AE, et al. Differences in inducibility and prognosis of in-hospital versus out-of-hospital identified nonsustained ventricular tachycardia in patients with coronary artery disease: clinical and trial design implications11For a complete list of participants see refer. J Am Coll Cardiol 2001; 38(4):1156–62.

23. Wit AL, Rosen MR. Pathophysiologic mechanisms of cardiac arrhythmias. Am Heart J 1983;106(4):798–811.

24. Cherry EM, Fenton FH, Gilmour RF. Mechanisms of ventricular arrhythmias: a dynamical systems-based perspective. Am J Physiol Circ Physiol 2012; 302(12):H2451–63.

25. Littmann L, Gibbs MA. Electrocardiographic manifestations of severe hyperkalemia. J Electrocardiol 2018;51(5):814–7.

26. Hollowell H, Mattu A, Perron AD, et al. Wide-complex tachycardia: beyond the traditional differential diagnosis of ventricular tachycardia vs supraventricular tachycardia with aberrant conduction. Am J Emerg Med 2005;23(7):876–89.

27. Garner JB, Miller JM. Wide Complex Tachycardia – Ventricular Tachycardia or Not Ventricular Tachycardia, that remains the question. Arrhythmia Electrophysiol Rev 2013;2(1):23.

28. Littmann L, Olson EG, Gibbs MA. Initial evaluation and management of wide-complex tachycardia: a simplified and practical approach. Am J Emerg Med 2019. https://doi.org/10.1016/j.ajem.2019.04.027.

29. May AM, Brenes-Salazar JA, DeSimone CV, et al. Electrocardiogram algorithms used to differentiate wide complex tachycardias demonstrate diagnostic limitations when applied by non-cardiologists. J Electrocardiol 2018;51(6):1103–9.

30. Trohman RG, Parrillo JE. Direct current cardioversion: Indications, techniques, and recent advances. Crit Care Med 2000;28(Supplement):N170–3.

31. Ortiz M, Martín A, Arribas F, et al. Randomized comparison of intravenous procainamide vs. intravenous amiodarone for the acute treatment of tolerated wide QRS tachycardia: the PROCAMIO study. Eur Heart J 2016. https://doi.org/10.1093/eurheartj/ehw230. ehw230.

32. Marill KA, Wolfram S, DeSouza IS, et al. Adenosine for wide-complex tachycardia: Efficacy and safety. Crit Care Med 2009;37(9):2512–8.

33. Goldberger ZD, Rho RW, Page RL. Approach to the Diagnosis and Initial Management of the Stable Adult Patient With a Wide Complex Tachycardia. Am J Cardiol 2008;101(10):1456–66.

Emergency Department Evaluation and Management of Patients with Left Ventricular Assist Devices

Akilesh Honasoge, MD[a], Kami M. Hu, MD[b,c],*

KEYWORDS

- Congestive heart failure • CHF • Left ventricular assist device • LVAD • HeartMate
- HeartWare • HVAD • Mechanical circulatory devices

KEY POINTS

- The rapid assessment of a patient with aleft ventricular assist device(LVAD) includes quick determination of "sick" versus "not sick" and evaluation of LVAD components, parameters, and alarms.
- Common complications include stroke, hemorrhage, driveline infection, device thrombus or failure, arrhythmias, and right ventricular (RV) failure.
- Recognition of alarm implications and use of bedside echocardiography can quickly narrow the differential if the diagnosis is not immediately evident.
- Initial stabilization includes ensuring appropriate LVAD functioning, volume resuscitation when indicated, and often the same pathology-targeted treatments as in patients without LVADs.

INTRODUCTION

Congestive heart failure (CHF) is one of the most common comorbidities in patients presenting to the emergency department (ED), with more than 6.1 million ED patients in 2019 carrying a diagnosis of CHF.[1] As a patient's heart failure progresses, they may become a candidate for certain advanced therapies including a left ventricular assist device (LVAD), a surgically implanted device that actively removes blood from the left ventricle and delivers it to the aorta. The growth in prevalence of these mechanical

[a] Department of Internal Medicine, Division of Cardiology, Rush Medical College, 600 South Paulina Street, Chicago, IL 60612, USA; [b] Department of Emergency, University of Maryland School of Medicine, 110 South Paca Street, 6th Floor, Suite 200, Baltimore, MD 21201, USA; [c] Department of Internal Medicine, University of Maryland School of Medicine, 110 South Paca Street, 6th Floor, Suite 200, Baltimore, MD 21201, USA
* Corresponding author. Department of Emergency Medicine, University of Maryland School of Medicine, 110 South Paca Street, 6th Floor, Suite 200, Baltimore, MD 21201.
E-mail address: khu@som.umaryland.edu

Emerg Med Clin N Am 40 (2022) 755–770
https://doi.org/10.1016/j.emc.2022.06.011
0733-8627/22/© 2022 Elsevier Inc. All rights reserved.
emed.theclinics.com

devices means that patients with an LVAD may present to any ED for both cardiac and noncardiac complaints. Although an intimate understanding of LVAD function is limited for most physicians, LVADs are conceptually simple devices. A basic understanding of LVAD mechanics, as well as familiarity with the common causes of decompensation in this patient population, provides a much more straightforward approach to the management of these patients when acutely ill.

BACKGROUND
Indications for Left Ventricular Assist Device Therapy

As patients progress in severity toward end-stage heart failure they may undergo the evaluation of candidacy for advanced therapies, with heart transplantation being the ultimate therapy. With a median posttransplant survival of 10.7 years, few other modalities come close to this target in patients with end-stage heart failure.[2] Due to the scarcity of heart donors and delays in finding a suitable match, many transplant candidates require mechanical support as a bridge to transplant (BTT). In comparison to other mechanical circulatory support options such as extracorporeal membrane oxygenation (ECMO), the modern LVAD allows the patient to live at home with survival rates greater than a year from implantation. LVADs may be used as destination therapy (DT) instead of BTT for patients who are poor candidates for heart transplantation.

While multiple companies and devices exist, emergency providers need only be familiar with three: the HeartMate II (Thoratec/St. Jude/Abbott), HVAD (HeartWare/Medtronic), and HeartMate 3 (Abbott) (**Fig. 1**). The HeartMate II device is the oldest device still widely used due to its long history of proven results and predictable complications and is approved for both BTT and DT. The HVAD was also approved for both BTT and DT[3] until June 2021 when the US Food and Drug Administration issued a Class I recall due to an increased risk of neurologic adverse events and higher pump failure rates.[4] Given the risk and morbidity associated with explantation, numerous patients remain implanted with an HVAD and are still supported by Medtronic. The HeartMate 3 is the most recently approved device for both BTT and long-term therapy and is now the most commonly implanted LVAD.[5]

Left Ventricular Assist Device Components and Function

Continuous-flow devices have become the standard of care given their advantages over pulsatile pumps which includes smaller size, reduced noise and energy use,

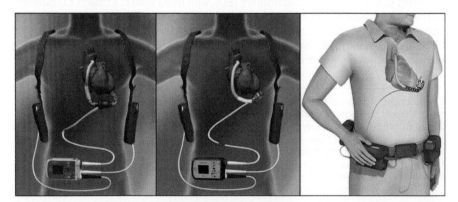

Fig. 1. Current widely used left-ventricular assist devices, from left to right: the HeartMate II, HeartMate 3, and HeartWare HVAD. *Courtesy* of Abbott and Medtronic. HeartMate II and HeartMate 3 are trademarks of Abbott or its related companies. Reproduced with permission of Abbott, © 2022. All rights reserved.

fewer moving parts, and less surface area in contact with blood resulting in fewer points of thrombogenesis and impaired flow.[6] The two main types of continuous flow pumps include the older axial flow pump used by the HeartMate II and the newer centrifugal flow pump outfitted in the HVAD and HeartMate 3. Centrifugal pumps require significantly less rotational speed than axial pumps to achieve the same energy transfer and blood flow rates, thus requiring less power and exerting less shear stress on blood cells, with less heat production and lower rates of hemolysis.[7]

The LVAD is completely contained within the patient's body apart from the driveline, a coated electrical wire that exits the body to connect the LVAD to the system controller and external power source. Component functions are listed in **Table 1**. The inflow graft of the LVAD is positioned at the LV apex to aim toward the mitral valve and minimize interaction with the interventricular septum[8] and the outflow graft is positioned on the proximal ascending aorta.[9] The system controller allows rapid review of the LVAD parameters and alarms, especially if a model-specific LVAD system monitor is not readily available (**Fig. 2**). The HeartMate II and HeartMate 3 each have a "display" button, that when pressed cycles through the display of the LVAD settings and battery charge status. When pressed simultaneously with the "silence alarm" button, the last 6 alarms can be reviewed.[10,11] Similarly, pressing the "scroll" button on the HVAD controller will allow the review of pump parameters and alarms.

Left Ventricular Assist Device Parameters and Physiology

Long-term LVAD management and setting optimization can be a complex process, but the ED management of LVADs relies on a basic interpretation of previously established LVAD parameters (**Table 2**), general cardiac hemodynamics, and device alarm interpretation.

A key concept in LVAD physiology is the differential or "head pressure" (ΔP), the difference in pressure between the aortic outflow cannula and the LV inflow cannula.[12]

$$\Delta P = \text{aortic pressure - left ventricular pressure}$$

With an increase in ΔP there is a higher gradient of pressure for the LVAD to pump across. This results in decreased LVAD flow as the speed is a set parameter that remains the same. In diastole, the LV pressure decreases, resulting in increased ΔP, decreased LVAD flow, and less power required to maintain the set speed. Conversely, during systole the contracting LV increases LV pressure and lowers the ΔP, thereby

Table 1	
LVAD components and their functions	
Component	**Function**
Pump	Actively takes blood from the LV via the inflow cannula and pumps it into the aorta via the outflow cannula HeartMate II pump sits in a preperitoneal pocket HeartMate 3 and HVAD sit at the LV apex
Driveline	Travels percutaneously to connect the internal pump to the external system controller and power supply
System Controller	Continuously monitors pump function and performance Displays LVAD battery status, device metrics, and alarms
Power Supply	Electricity source for the device; includes batteries for travel and power station that plus directly into the wall

Abbreviations: HVAD, HeartWare continuous flow ventricular assist device; LV, left ventricle; LVAD, left ventricular assist device.

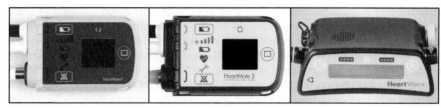

Fig. 2. HeartMate II, HeartMate 3, and HeartWare System Controllers (in order from left to right;). *Courtesy* of Abbott and Medtronic. HeartMate II and HeartMate 3 are trademarks of Abbott or its related companies. Reproduced with permission of Abbott, © 2022. All rights reserved.

increasing the flow across the device as well as the compensatory power required to maintain the set speed. This example highlights how a heart with a continuous-flow LVAD still retains elements of pulsatile flow, how the resultant power fluctuations can allow the LVAD to quantify said pulsatility, and why the pulsatility of LVAD flow at a given programmed speed is an indicator of native LV contribution to cardiac output. High pulsatility occurs with greater native LV contribution, whether due to increased LV function, hypervolemia, or issues resulting in decreased relative pump contribution. Low pulsatility indicates that most of the output is being provided by the LVAD, either due to decreased LV filling, worsened native LV function, or increased LVAD flows due to processes such as systemic vasodilation that lower the ΔP.[12]

Pump pulsatility is measured and displayed differently based on the LVAD type. The HeartMate II and HeartMate 3 pumps display a single number called the pulsatility index (PI), a unitless number that measures the beat-to-beat variability of the pump power use as averaged over 10 to 15 seconds.

$$PI = \frac{maximum\ power - minimum\ power}{average\ power}$$

Table 2
LVAD settings and hemodynamic parameters

Metric	Units	Definition	Additional Information
Speed	RPM	Rate of pump rotation	Set by LVAD engineer based on echocardiographic ramp study[13] Remains relatively constant if device functioning properly
Power	Watts	Amount of energy required to achieve set speed	Variable depending on device and patient characteristics Responds to change in flow to maintain speed (lower flows require less power)
Flow	L/min	Estimated LVAD output	Calculated by LVAD using speed, power, and blood viscosity[11,13] Proportional to Speed, Inversely proportional to ΔP (therefore preload dependent, afterload sensitive)
Pulsatility Index (PI)	N/A	An indirect measure of native LV function and preload contribution to cardiac output	Higher PI indicates more contribution from preload/native LV contraction and less from the LVAD itself.

Abbreviations: ΔP, differential pressure; L/min, liters per minute; LV, left ventricle; LVAD, left ventricular assist device; RPM, revolutions per minute.

Of note, the HeartMate 3 has a special "artificial pulse" setting with alternating speeds designed to minimize stasis, which adds extra pulsatility to the continuous flow LVAD.[11,12] Alternately, the HVAD displays a real-time waveform of pump flow on the system monitor, the amplitude of which is a measure of pulsatility,[12] correlated to native LV contribution to output and therefore inversely correlated to the amount of output the LVAD must provide.

Left Ventricular Assist Device Alarm Significance

System controller review instructions and descriptions of possible alarms can be found on the manufacturer's websites. Alarms denoting low battery or driveline failure quickly narrow whereby the difficulty may lie. Similarly, recognition of other alarm patterns narrows the differential for causative pathology, as most of the LVAD-associated illnesses can be delineated by first determining whether LVAD flow is high or low, then assessing for increased or decreased pulsatility (**Fig. 3**). Power is usually proportional to speed and flow, but a high power alarm in the setting of normal or even low flow indicates pump thrombus, as more energy must be applied to maintain speed. The HVAD has a specific alarm for suction events, when the near-complete collapse of the LV leads to the wall being sucked into the inflow cannula. LVADs intentionally drop speed when suction events occur or are impending, so these events are manifested as low-speed alarms without battery or power failure in the HeartMate II and 3. Very importantly, critical alarms indicating ongoing or impending device failure will sound continuously on any system controller, indicating the need for immediate attention.

Emergency Department Evaluation of Patients with a Left Ventricular Assist Device

The arrival of an LVAD patient to the ED should prompt the notification of the patient's LVAD coordinator, especially in resource-limited settings without the ability to provide the full spectrum of care required. They are usually familiar with baseline LVAD parameters for the patient, can help with alarm interpretation, and may also be able to provide medical history or help coordinate transfer.

The ABCDE's

The initial evaluation of patients with LVAD is essentially the same as for any other patient, with the inclusion of specific components that can be remembered using the "ABCDE" mnemonic (**Table 3**). If these components are reassuring, the patient is less likely to be critically ill and additional ED workup can proceed as usual.

Table 3		
The ABCDE of rapid LVAD patient evaluation		
A	Appearance	Alert, Normal Skin Perfusion
	Auscultation	Smooth hum of Working Device
B	Battery	Charged and connected to the power source
	Blood Pressure	MAP 70–90 mm Hg
C	Controller	No alarms
		Not hot to touch
		Device metrics unchanged
D	Driveline	Externally intact, no signs of damage or infection
E	Echocardiogram	Baseline LV:RV ratio, no tamponade or LV underfilling
	ECG	Normal sinus rhythm, rate-controlled arrhythmia

Abbreviations: ECG, electrocardiogram; LV, left ventricle; MAP, mean arterial pressure; RV, right ventricle.

Appearance and auscultation

Altered mentation and mottled skin or poor capillary refill are worrisome signs of poor end-organ perfusion and potential severe LVAD malfunction. A quick check with the stethoscope should confirm the smooth hum of a working LVAD impeller.

Battery and blood pressure

Prompt evaluation of the battery not only identifies potential issues but can preempt decompensation, as it is important that the LVAD remain connected to a power source. Recognition of abnormal blood pressure can quickly identify a target for treatment as patients with LVAD are preload-dependent and afterload-sensitive with a narrow range for the goal MAP, with guidelines supporting a target between 70 and 80 mm Hg.[13,14] Standard automatic noninvasive blood pressure cuff assessments are often either unobtainable or inaccurate in patients with LVADs, many of whom may not actually have a detectable pulse. The gold standard blood pressure assessment is obtained via an arterial line,[15] although this may not be practical in the ED setting. Ideal noninvasive measurement of an LVAD patient's blood pressure involves

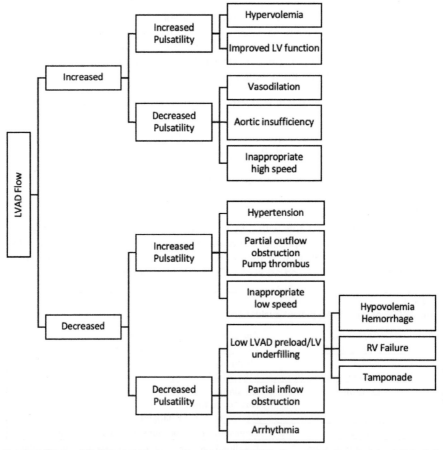

Fig. 3. Differential diagnosis for causes of altered LVAD flow. LV, left ventricle; LVAD, left ventricular assist device; RV, right ventricle. (*Data from* [Tchoukina I, Smallfield MC, Shah KB. Device Management and Flow Optimization on Left Ventricular Assist Device Support. Crit Care Clin. 2018;34(3):453-463].)

inflating a manual arm cuff and then slowly deflating it, assessing for blood flow using doppler ultrasound.[16] The first evidence of flow heard is generally denoted as the mean arterial pressure (MAP) as the patient's pulsatility is often too low to accurately parse out the difference between systolic and diastolic pressure.[16]

Connections and controller alarms
Ensure all connections between the battery, controller, and driveline are intact and check the system controller for logged alarms and settings. There are a variety of self-explanatory alarms (eg, low battery charge or driveline disconnection) but as stated above, alarms for flow or pulsatility changes generally indicate an issue that will require intervention.

Driveline
Confirm that the driveline is externally intact and check the abdominal wall entry site for signs of infection. If there is a concern for internal driveline fracture or driveline-associated infection, further evaluation with X-rays or computed tomography scan should be pursued.

Echocardiography and electrocardiogram
For sick patients with an LVAD, bedside "echo" is a quick and helpful tool to narrow the differential diagnosis and guide management. While it may be difficult to get all the expected cardiac views, the most important assessment is the appearance of the ventricles, particularly the left. LV systolic function is expected to be poor but understanding the relative size of the ventricles will help guide ED diagnosis (**Fig. 4**).[14]

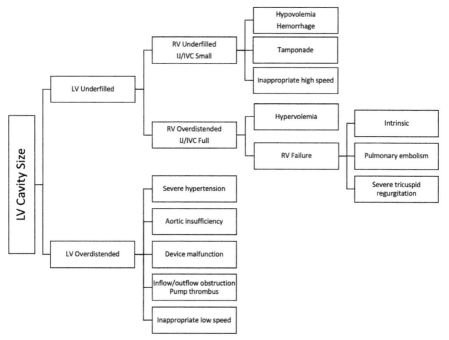

Fig. 4. Differential for LVAD complications based on point-of-care echocardiography. IJ, internal jugular vein; IVC, inferior vena cava; LV, left ventricle; RV, right ventricle.

All patients with an LVAD require an electrocardiogram (ECG) for the evaluation of heart rate and rhythm.[14] Although arrhythmias are relatively well-tolerated in patients with LVADs,[17] a physical examination is typically insufficient to detect these as the loud LVAD hum and the lack of regular valve opening and closing make auscultation unreliable and peripheral pulsatility may be too low for assessment.

Additional Diagnostic Considerations

Basic bloodwork should be obtained on all patients with LVADs, with additional lab testing as indicated by diagnostic concern based on patient presentation and LVAD alarm review **(Table 4)**. As traditional pulse oximetry relies on pulsatility, accurate oxygenation assessment in an LVAD patient may require an arterial blood gas if there is a concern for hypoxemia. X-ray imaging can be useful to estimate appropriate device positioning and assess for driveline fracture or kinking while simultaneously evaluating for other non-LVAD pathologies. Computed tomography (CT) can be used to further assess driveline integrity but also identifies fluid collections, device thrombosis, heart chamber size, and pericardial effusions. As previously discussed, the emergency physician's most useful imaging tool for LVAD assessment remains point-of-care echocardiography.

Table 4
Initial emergency department workup for patients with LVAD

Diagnostic Concern	Laboratories	Imaging	Other
Basic Work-Up	Complete blood count Comprehensive metabolic panel Prothrombin/INR Partial prothrombin time Lactate (if critically ill)	Consider chest/ abdomen x-ray	ECG Consider echo
Primary Cardiac Issue	Troponin Brain natriuretic peptide	Chest x-ray	Echo
Anemia/Hemorrhage	Lactate dehydrogenase Plasma-free hemoglobin Fibrinogen Consider thromboelastogram	Consider abdominal CTA	Echo FAST
LVAD Malfunction or Obstruction	All of the above	Chest and abdomen x-ray CT chest with IV contrast	Echo
Infection	Blood cultures Urinalysis with reflex culture Other cultures as appropriate (including driveline site)	Chest x-ray Consider CT chest/ abdomen with IV contrast	

Abbreviations: CT(A), computed tomography(angiography); ECG, electrocardiogram; FAST, focused assessment with sonography in trauma; INR, international normalized ratio; IV, intravenous.

EMERGENT LEFT VENTRICULAR ASSIST DEVICE COMPLICATIONS

Recognition of the life-threatening complications for which patients with LVADs are at risk is crucial to help guide the emergency physician in asking the right questions, obtaining appropriate diagnostics, and achieving stabilization in the ED. One helpful mnemonic, "DEATHS," is outlined in **Table 5**.

Table 5 DEATHS mnemonic for potentially life-threatening LVAD emergencies	
D	Driveline Complications (Fracture, infection) Device Failure
E	Embolism (ischemic stroke)
A	Arrhythmia (atrial, ventricular)
T	Thrombus (device)
H	Hemorrhage (GI, epistaxis, intracranial, pericardial)
S	Suckdown

Abbreviation: GI, gastrointestinal.

Left Ventricular Assist Device-Specific Complications

Driveline fracture

Although data are somewhat limited, the rate of postimplantation driveline fracture is thought to be relatively low.[18] Fractures may or may not be readily evident and patients may present asymptomatic or mildly symptomatic with controller alarms indicating driveline malfunction or low voltage, decreased speed/power, or low flow — or they may present in extremis with pump arrest. Patients with suspected driveline fractures should undergo anterior–posterior and lateral chest and abdominal x-rays. Confirmed fractures require emergent cardiac surgery consultation, with inotropes made available while arranging transfer to the nearest LVAD facility, as the nonsurgical management options are limited.[18]

Device infections

Infections can be classified as LVAD-specific, LVAD-related, and non-LVAD. LVAD-specific infections include infections of the device itself, either driveline or surgical pocket infections. Driveline infections are the most common LVAD-specific infection, and external signs of driveline site infection should prompt the collection of blood cultures and a contrasted CT of the chest and abdomen to determine the extent of infection. The most common pathogens causing LVAD-specific infections are shown in **Table 6**.[19] Mild, superficial infections can most often be treated with appropriate gram-positive coverage of skin flora, while more severe or deeper infections should include coverage for methicillin-resistant Staphylococcus aureus and gram-negative coverage with antipseudomonal activity.[19] Deep driveline infections involving the fascia or muscles may require operative debridement, extended antibiotic therapy. Infections extending to the device itself, as well as LVAD-related infections such as bacteremia, endocarditis, and mediastinitis are also treated with prolonged antibiotics, often requiring intraoperative debridement and cultures to appropriately narrow antimicrobial therapy.[19] Non–LVAD-related infections such as pneumonia or urinary tract infections can become more difficult to treat as patients are often already on suppressive antibiotics, and minimizing unnecessary indwelling devices such as central venous and urinary catheters is key. LVAD-associated infections should, in most instances, prompt admission to the hospital for treatment in consultation with an infectious disease specialist given the variety of indwelling hardware, historical exposure to numerous antibiotics, and the high morbidity associated with an undertreated infection.[19] It is important to be cognizant of possible antimicrobial drug interactions, as most patients with LVADs are on warfarin.

Table 6 Causative organisms in LVAD-specific infections	
Organisms	Frequency
Staphylococcus (aureus and epidermidis)	>50%
Enterococcus	2%
Pseudomonas aeruginosa	22%–28%
Klebsiella	2%–4%
Enterobacter	2%
Candida (albicans and glabrata)	1.3%–9.7%

Pump thrombosis

All patients with a continuous-flow LVAD should be taking daily low-dose aspirin and therapeutic warfarin with an international normalized ratio (INR) goal of 2 to 3, although the goal may be adjusted based on patient-specific complication history.[13] Despite strict compliance to this regimen and advancements in technology, device thrombosis can still occur near the impeller as well as in the inflow or outflow grafts, carrying the potential for secondary embolic complications. Pump thrombosis should be suspected in the presence of acute heart failure symptoms with low flow alarms or increased power use.[20] A CT scan may suggest or confirm possible device thrombosis, but the primary initial method of diagnosis is via bloodwork. A serum lactate dehydrogenase (LDH) level > 2.5 times the upper limit of normal carries a relatively high sensitivity (78%) and specificity (97%) for pump thrombosis,[21] although the diagnosis is usually confirmed with plasma-free hemoglobin. Decreased haptoglobin levels are common due to continuously low levels of hemolysis, and do not necessarily indicate pump thrombosis.[20,21]

The medical management of device thrombosis can vary depending on the patient's clinical status and findings on echocardiography with a ramp study, ranging from an increase in antiplatelet therapy to increased anticoagulation to even potentially intravenous or catheter-directed thrombolytics. In extreme circumstances whereby medical therapy fails to improve a patient's pump thrombosis or hemolysis, a surgical pump exchange or expedited heart transplant is considered.[20,21]

Device failure/cardiac arrest

Cardiac arrest may occur either due to or independently of device failure. As pulselessness is unreliable, unresponsiveness with agonal or absent respirations should be treated as presumed or impending arrest until otherwise determined. Despite historical concerns about device dislodgment, cardiopulmonary resuscitation with chest compressions should be started immediately[22] with concurrent attempts to notify the patient's VAD team.

If the device is powered on, as evidenced by the detection of a device hum on chest auscultation, standard ACLS resuscitative measures to restore effective circulation should be pursued while evaluating the device components and performing bedside echo per the ABCDE assessment. A loud, continuous controller alarm should prompt immediate attention as it likely indicates impending or active LVAD failure. The absence of device hum on auscultation confirms failure and the need to restart the

LVAD (**Table 7**). If none of these measures are effective in restarting the LVAD, attempts to restore circulation via standard ACLS resuscitation efforts should be trialed. Even in the setting of a functioning LVAD, CPR is recommended if there is evidence of poor perfusion such as a MAP $\leq$50 mm Hg or partial pressure of end-tidal carbon dioxide (PETCO$_2$) $\leq$20 mm Hg from an endotracheal tube.[22]

If the patient arrests at a hospital with ECMO capability, emergent consultation for extracorporeal life support (ECLS) may be reasonable in patients listed for cardiac transplant depending on specific patient factors.

Table 7 Troubleshooting LVAD failure in cardiac arrest[23]		
Power Failure	Step 1	Check that External LVAD Components are Intact and Appropriately Connected.
	Step 2	Ensure the LVAD is hooked up to a working power source • Check battery charge by pressing the button on the physical battery • Transition to wall power if needed
If the LVAD does not restart after Steps 1 and 2, proceed to Step 3		
Controller Failure	Step 3	Connect the patient's spare system controller to a charged battery or wall power, then switch the driveline's connection to the spare controller
If the LVAD does not restart after Step 3, proceed to Step 4		
Internal Driveline Fracture	Step 4	Gently manipulate the driveline to see if manual "reconnection" of an internal fracture can restart the LVAD.
	Step 5	If the LVAD restarts, stabilize the driveline in the appropriate position with tape

Abbreviation: LVAD, left ventricular assist device.

Left Ventricular Assist Device-Associated Complications

Neurologic events

Strokes are often devastating in patients with LVADs, not only due to the increase in morbidity and mortality but due to the potential impact on heart transplant candidacy.[24] Patients with LVADs are at a higher risk of ischemic and hemorrhagic stroke with an estimated rate of 7%, 11%, and 17% at 6, 12, and 24 months, respectively, after LVAD implantation.[25] Factors such as increased age, history of diabetes, infection, and prior stroke history increase a patient's risk, and uncontrolled hypertension with a systolic blood pressure >100 mm Hg increases stroke risk by 2.5 times.[26] Management of a hemorrhagic stroke often involves neurosurgical consultation and anticoagulation reversal with vitamin K and possibly prothrombin complex concentrate (PCC). Management of an ischemic stroke is limited as the patients are typically already fully anticoagulated, decreasing their candidacy for thrombolytics.[27]

Arrythmias

Arrythmias are extremely common in patients with LVADs[17] due to a combination of the underlying myocardial disease and significant electrical disruption from the device itself. ECG interpretation of arrhythmias can be difficult due to the significant artifact from the LVAD. Fortunately, most arrythmias are well-tolerated both symptomatically and hemodynamically as the patient's cardiac output is not reliant on left ventricular function itself.[17] Bedside echocardiography can be helpful to guide therapy, as cardiac chambers that are both over and under-distended can increase myocardial irritability. If the LV and right ventricular (RV) are underfilled and/or the IVC is collapsible, the administration of fluids may help improve the heart rate while a clearly distended LV, especially if there are other signs of hypervolemia, will need diuresis to help adequately manage the arrhythmia.

Preexisting atrial arrhythmias (AA) are found in up to 54% of patients' preimplantation, while de novo AA after LVAD implantation occurs in anywhere from 20% to 30%.[17] Due to a paucity of data, there is no clear benefit to pursuing rhythm control over rate control or vice versa, and long-term management should be specifically tailored to the patient by his or her cardiologist. For the euvolemic LVAD patient presenting to the ED with a rapid ventricular rate (RVR) and stable MAP and LVAD flows, rate control can be initially attempted with beta-blockers and/or digoxin, with the addition of amiodarone as a next step for refractory RVR. In cases of AA with RVR causing clear extremis, electrical cardioversion should be promptly performed.[17,28]

Ventricular arrhythmias are generally well-tolerated in patients with an LVAD. The most common symptoms are palpitations, fatigue, and presyncope,[29] but both ventricular tachycardia (VT) and ventricular fibrillation (VF) can even be asymptomatic. Symptoms and decreased LVAD flows occur secondary to poor RV function during arrhythmia leading to decreased LV filling. Left ventricular function is often not significantly affected if the LVAD itself is still functioning properly. Antiarrhythmics and beta-blockers are still primary therapies but have not been shown to improve morbidity and mortality.[29] Cardioversion and defibrillation are reasonable options, safe, and should be performed in patients with LVAD who are extremely symptomatic despite medical therapy.[17,29]

Gastrointestinal hemorrhage

Continuous-flow LVADs are associated with a significant increase in the incidence of hemorrhage, including epistaxis, intracranial hemorrhage, and gastrointestinal (GI) bleeding. In fact, it is the most common complication after LVAD implantation.[30] This increase is likely in part related to the concurrent use of antiplatelet and anticoagulant therapy, but when compared with patients with a mechanical valve replacement on similar regimens, patients with LVADs still have a higher rate of bleeding.[30,31] This increased risk is theorized to be due to the increased shear stresses on blood leading to impaired platelet aggregation and an acquired von Willebrand Syndrome, as well as a reduced pulse pressure leading to the formation of angiodysplastic lesions.[30]

Bleeding can occur anywhere along the GI tract but upper GI bleeds are most common (47%).[32] While AVMs are the most commonly identified etiology (up to 44%), additional causes include gastritis (22%), peptic ulcer disease (13%), and diverticular hemorrhage (6%) among others.[32] The medical management of LVAD-related bleeding is similar to that of non–LVAD-related bleeding. Hemodynamic stabilization with blood product transfusion is of utmost importance, with a frequent reassessment of the patient including serial bedside echocardiography to help guide transfusion.

Anticoagulation reversal in this setting is controversial, but many advocates for the reversal of warfarin with vitamin K, and some recommend the use of prothrombin complex concentrate (PCC).[32] Data are limited[33] but PCC administration carries a risk of LVAD device thrombosis and subsequent stroke, both potentially catastrophic consequences. Further medical therapies include the use of a proton pump inhibitor for presumed upper GI bleeding and consideration of octreotide for splanchnic vaso-constriction, as well as desmopressin to maximize the availability of von Willebrand factor.[32]

Endoscopy remains a mainstay of management, usually after initial stabilization. If the source of the bleed is not found or emergent GI consultation is unavailable on-site, additional ED workup may be performed with CT angiography while transfer to another facility is being arranged. The persistently unstable patient with GI bleed who fails endoscopic therapy should also prompt consideration for a consultation with an interventional radiologist for endovascular management.

Suction events

A suction, or "suckdown," event is caused by a transient obstruction of the inflow can-nula, usually due to an underfilled left ventricle that collapses such that the LV wall gets "sucked in" to the inflow cannula causing a temporary blockage of blood flow.[13] LVADs are programmed to identify impending suction events by recognizing abrupt changes to the PI, and in response, the LVAD drops the device speed temporarily down to the lowest functional speed to decrease LV emptying and thereby increase the LV chamber size before ramping back up to the normal speed.[10,11] This adjust-ment can happen transiently when a patient is moving from a seated to standing po-sition too quickly or the patient performs a Valsalva maneuver. Recurrent alarms, however, should clue emergency providers into a dangerously underfilled LV that can be quickly identified on bedside echo.[13] Causes of LV underfilling and therefore suction events include RV failure, tamponade, severe hypovolemia, or less likely, inap-propriate set speed.

Right ventricular failure

Many patients with left ventricular dysfunction severe enough to require an LVAD have some element of RV dysfunction, and up to 40% of patients develop RV failure in the weeks after LVAD implantation.[34] This RV failure is often reversible, but for patients in whom it is not clinical management is challenging. Medical management includes ino-tropes, pulmonary vasodilators, diuretics, and decreasing pump speed. If these mea-sures are unsuccessful, the patient will need to be considered for a RV assist device (RVAD), total artificial heart (TAH), other forms of mechanical support, or a palliative approach.[21]

SUMMARY

The care of a patient with an LVAD may seem daunting but is actually relatively formu-laic. Systematically yet rapidly assessing the patient's perfusion and LVAD compo-nents quickly identifies the need for emergent interventions. The review of alarms and bedside echocardiography, in addition to relevant diagnostics and ECG, allows the emergency physician to focus on the likely diagnosis and take steps to address the underlying pathology.

CLINICS CARE POINTS

- Contacting the patient's VAD coordinator early in the ED course can expedite appropriate care, as they are familiar with the patient and can help facilitate transfer if needed.

- Evaluation of an LVAD should always include: ensuring the device is on and appropriately powered, that all parts are intact and well-connected, and that any alarms are reviewed.

- LVADs are preload-dependent and afterload-sensitive. Maintenance/restoration of euvolemia and strict blood pressure control is key to maintaining normal device output.
- Arrhythmias are usually well-tolerated and should be managed with the restoration of euvolemia if needed and standard medical therapies or cardioversion/defibrillation as appropriate.
- Chest compressions are not contraindicated in cardiac arrest and should not be withheld out of concern for device dislodgement.

DISCLOSURE

The authors have no financial disclosures or conflicts of interest.

REFERENCES

1. Cairns C, Kang K. National Hospital Ambulatory Medical Care Survey: 2019 emergency department summary tables. 2022. Available at: https://www.cdc.gov/nchs/data/nhamcs/web_tables/2019-nhamcs-ed-web-tables-508.pdf. Accessed May 5, 2022.
2. Lund LH, Khush KK, Cherikh WS, et al. The registry of the international society for heart and lung transplantation: thirty-fourth adult heart transplantation report—2017; focus theme: allograft ischemic time. J Heart Lung Transpl 2017;36(10):1037–46.
3. Stehlik J, Kirklin JK. The long and winding road to an effective left ventricular assist device: the demise of medtronic's HVAD. Circulation 2021;144(7):509–11.
4. US Food and Drug Administration. Stop new implants of the medtronic HVAD system – letter to health care providers. 2021. Available at: https://www.fda.gov/medical-devices/letters-health-care-providers/stop-new-implants-medtronic-hvad-system-letter-health-care-providers. Accessed January 9, 2022.
5. Molina EJ, Shah P, Kiernan MS, et al. The society of thoracic surgeons intermacs 2020 annual report. Ann Thorac Surg 2021;111(3):778–92.
6. Kato TS, Chokshi A, Singh P, et al. Effects of continuous-flow versus pulsatile-flow left ventricular assist devices on myocardial unloading and remodeling. Circ Heart Fail 2011;4(5):546–53.
7. Tchoukina I, Smallfield MC, Shah KB. Device management and flow optimization on left ventricular assist device support. Crit Care Clin 2018;34(3):453–63.
8. Stulak JM, Abou El Ela A, Pagani FD. Implantation of a durable left ventricular assist device: how i teach it. Ann Thorac Surg 2017;103(6):1687–92.
9. Whitson BA. Surgical implant techniques of left ventricular assist devices: an overview of acute and durable devices. J Thorac Dis 2015;7(12):2097–101.
10. Thoratec Abbott. HeartMate II left ventricular assist system instructions for use featuring the mobile power unit. 2020. Available at: https://manuals.sjm.com/. Accessed January 30, 2022.
11. Thoratec Abbott. HeartMate 3 left ventricular assist system instructions for use with system monitor II. Available at: https://manuals.sjm.com/. Accessed January 30, 2022.
12. Belkin MN, Kagan V, Labuhn C, et al. Physiology and clinical utility of heartmate pump parameters. J Card Fail 2022;28(5):845–62. Published online December 2021:S1071916421004814.

13. Feldman D, Pamboukian SV, Teuteberg JJ, et al. The 2013 international society for heart and lung transplantation guidelines for mechanical circulatory support: executive summary. J Heart Lung Transpl 2013;32(2):157–87.

14. Givertz MM, DeFilippis EM, Colvin M, et al. HFSA/SAEM/ISHLT clinical expert consensus document on the emergency management of patients with ventricular assist devices. J Heart Lung Transpl 2019;38(7):677–98.

15. Bennett MK, Roberts CA, Dordunoo D, et al. Ideal methodology to assess systemic blood pressure in patients with continuous-flow left ventricular assist devices. J Heart Lung Transpl 2010;29(5):593–4.

16. Lanier GM, Orlanes K, Hayashi Y, et al. Validity and reliability of a novel slow cuff-deflation system for noninvasive blood pressure monitoring in patients with continuous-flow left ventricular assist device. Circ Heart Fail 2013;6(5):1005–12.

17. Gopinathannair R, Cornwell WK, Dukes JW, et al. Device therapy and arrhythmia management in left ventricular assist device recipients: a scientific statement from the american heart association. Circulation 2019;139(20):e967–89.

18. D'Antonio ND, Maynes EJ, Tatum RT, et al. Driveline damage and repair in continuous-flow left ventricular assist devices: A systematic review. Artif Organs 2021;45(8):819–26.

19. Kusne S, Mooney M, Danziger-Isakov L, et al. An ISHLT consensus document for prevention and management strategies for mechanical circulatory support infection. J Heart Lung Transpl 2017;36(10):1137–53.

20. Goldstein DJ, John R, Salerno C, et al. Algorithm for the diagnosis and management of suspected pump thrombus. J Heart Lung Transpl 2013;32(7):667–70.

21. Kirklin JK, Pagani FD, Goldstein DJ, et al. American association for thoracic surgery/international society for heart and lung transplantation guidelines on selected topics in mechanical circulatory support. J Heart Lung Transpl 2020; 39(3):187–219.

22. Peberdy MA, Gluck JA, Ornato JP, et al. Cardiopulmonary resuscitation in adults and children with mechanical circulatory support: a scientific statement from the american heart association. Circulation 2017;135(24):e1115–34.

23. Bowles CT, Hards R, Wrightson N, et al. Algorithms to guide ambulance clinicians in the management of emergencies in patients with implanted rotary left ventricular assist devices. Emerg Med J 2017;34(12):842–50.

24. Cho SM, Moazami N, Frontera JA. Stroke and intracranial hemorrhage in heartmate ii and heartware left ventricular assist devices: a systematic review. Neurocrit Care 2017;27(1):17–25.

25. McNamara N, Narroway H, Williams M, et al. Contemporary outcomes of continuous-flow left ventricular assist devices-a systematic review. Ann Cardiothorac Surg 2021;10(2):186–208.

26. Nassif ME, Tibrewala A, Raymer DS, et al. Systolic blood pressure on discharge after left ventricular assist device insertion is associated with subsequent stroke. J Heart Lung Transpl 2015;34(4):503–8.

27. Al-Mufti F, Bauerschmidt A, Claassen J, et al. Neuroendovascular interventions for acute ischemic strokes in patients supported with left ventricular assist devices: a single-center case series and review of the literature. World Neurosurg 2016;88:199–204.

28. Ozcan C, Deshmukh A. Atrial arrhythmias in patients with left ventricular assist devices. Curr Opin Cardiol 2020;35(3):276–81.

29. Ahmed A, Amin M, Boilson BA, et al. Ventricular Arrhythmias in patients with left ventricular assist device (LVAD). Curr Treat Options Cardiovasc Med 2019; 21(11):75.

30. Shrode CW, Draper KV, Huang RJ, et al. Significantly higher rates of gastrointestinal bleeding and thromboembolic events with left ventricular assist devices. Clin Gastroenterol Hepatol 2014;12(9):1461–7.
31. Koyco A, Vural O, Bahcecitapar M, et al. Device-related epistaxis risk: continuous-flow left ventricular assist device-supported patients. Eur Arch Otorhinolaryngol 2020;277:2767–73.
32. Vedachalam S, Balasubramanian G, Haas GJ, et al. Treatment of gastrointestinal bleeding in left ventricular assist devices: A comprehensive review. World J Gastroenterol 2020;26(20):2550–8.
33. Jennings DL, Rimsans J, Connors JM. Prothrombin complex concentrate for warfarin reversal in patients with continuous-flow left ventricular assist devices: a narrative review. ASAIO J 2020;66(5):482–8.
34. Frankfurter C, Molinero M, Vishram-Nielsen JKK, et al. Predicting the risk of right ventricular failure in patients undergoing left ventricular assist device implantation: a systematic review. Circ Heart Fail 2020;13(10):e006994.

Cardiovascular Pharmacology

Jessica M. Mason, PharmD[a], Michael E. O'Brien, PharmD[a], Jennifer L. Koehl, PharmD[a], Christine S. Ji, PharmD[a], Bryan D. Hayes, PharmD[a,b,*]

KEYWORDS

- Cardiovascular • Pharmacology • Pharmacotherapy • Medication • Dosing
- Atrial fibrillation • Arrhythmia • Heart failure

KEY POINTS

- Terminology for defining acute coronary syndromes is shifting, but the initial pharmacotherapy for both ST-elevation and non-ST-elevation myocardial infarctions in the ED is similar.
- Critically ill acute heart failure patients generally require a combination of diuresis (loop diuretics) and preload reduction (vasodilation and/or noninvasive positive pressure ventilation). Cardiogenic shock patients may need vasopressors and inotropic support.
- Atrial fibrillation management can be complex and require multiple synergistic therapies including atrioventricular nodal blockade (calcium channel blockers or beta-blockers), magnesium, antiarrhythmics (eg, amiodarone, procainamide), and/or digoxin.
- Supraventricular tachycardia can be treated with adenosine or calcium channel blockers as the first-line options.
- For ventricular tachycardia and pulseless ventricular fibrillation, lidocaine or amiodarone can be administered. In refractory cases, esmolol should be considered.

INTRODUCTION

Pharmacologic therapy is an integral component in the management of most cardiovascular emergencies. This article reviews the pharmacotherapy involved in the treatment of acute coronary syndromes, acute heart failure (AHF) and cardiogenic shock (CS), and various arrhythmias including atrial fibrillation, supraventricular tachycardia (SVT), torsades de pointes (TdP), ventricular tachycardia/pulseless ventricular fibrillation (VF), and stable ventricular tachycardia. The goal is to provide practical pearls that can be

[a] Department of Pharmacy, Massachusetts General Hospital, 55 Fruit Street, Boston, MA 02114, USA; [b] Department of Emergency Medicine, Division of Medical Toxicology, Harvard Medical School, 55 Fruit Street, Boston, MA 02114, USA
* Corresponding author. Department of Pharmacy, Massachusetts General Hospital, 55 Fruit Street, Boston, MA 02114.
E-mail address: bryanhayes13@gmail.com
Twitter: @MikeEMPharmD (M.E.O.); @jlkoehl (J.L.K.); @PharmERToxGuy (B.D.H.)

Emerg Med Clin N Am 40 (2022) 771–792
https://doi.org/10.1016/j.emc.2022.06.012
0733-8627/22/© 2022 Elsevier Inc. All rights reserved.

applied at the bedside in the emergency department (ED). To provide clear takeaways for each type of emergency, this article is organized into succinct written sections and supplemented with comprehensive tables that include detailed drug information.

Acute Coronary Syndromes

Acute coronary syndrome (ACS) is an umbrella term encompassing non-ST-elevation ACS (NSTE-ACS), ST-elevation ACS (STE-ACS), and unstable angina. These syndromes are typically caused by an abrupt reduction in coronary blood flow resulting in myocardial ischemia or infarction; however, they are differentiated from each other based on the degree of vessel occlusion, electrocardiogram (ECG) changes, and presence/absence of cardiac biomarkers. New terminology for the classification of ACS was proposed encompassing occlusion MI and non-occlusion MI, rather than relying solely on ST-elevation as diagnostic criteria, in order to avoid missing an occlusive NSTE-ACS situation that would otherwise need immediate reperfusion.[1] This paradigm shift is not yet included in guidelines.

At the first point of medical contact in the ED, most patients with ACS are managed in the same way. This includes administration of oral (or rectal) aspirin as soon as feasible, nitroglycerin as needed for chest pain, and supplemental oxygen, if needed, to maintain O_2 saturation. If the patients are intolerant to aspirin or have an allergy, they should instead be loaded with a $P2Y_{12}$ inhibitor such as clopidogrel. Aspirin desensitization can be considered on admission. Additional pain control with opioids may be considered in patients whose chest pain is not relieved by nitroglycerin, though this is associated with worsened outcomes likely secondary to delayed absorption of antiplatelet agents.[2–5] Nonsteroidal anti-inflammatory drugs should be avoided in this clinical situation, as they can increase the risk of death and reinfarction.[6,7] Detailed information on the medications used in ACS can be found in **Table 1**.

ST-elevation-acute coronary syndrome

In patients with STE-ACS, immediate reperfusion with percutaneous coronary intervention (PCI) is preferred. In addition to initial aspirin, a $P2Y_{12}$ inhibitor and anticoagulation should be initiated as soon as possible either just before or during PCI. If PCI is not possible within 120 minutes, fibrinolytic therapy should be considered and initiated as soon as possible within 12 to 24 hours of symptom onset, ideally within 30 minutes of first medical contact. Guidelines prefer the use of fibrin-specific agents (eg, tenecteplase, alteplase, or reteplase) over streptokinase.[8,9]

Non-ST-elevation-acute coronary syndrome

In comparison, NSTE-ACS patients may be managed medically, with or without reperfusion. If PCI is performed, $P2Y_{12}$ inhibitors are typically initiated before or during PCI and are recommended to be continued for at least 12 months with aspirin.[10] Pretreatment with a $P2Y_{12}$ inhibitor (ticagrelor or clopidogrel) may be considered in NSTE-ACS patients before PCI; administration of prasugrel in patients with unknown coronary anatomy is not recommended. Anticoagulation, in addition to antiplatelet therapy, is recommended in all NSTE-ACS patients to be continued for the duration of hospital stay or until PCI.[11] It is important to note that anticoagulants only delay the onset of a potential cardiac event but do not modify underlying risk factors or physiology. Therefore, they may be best suited to patients who receive an intervention as the benefit does not persist following discontinuation or discharge.[12]

Other drug considerations

Statin therapy should be initiated in both NSTE-ACS and STE-ACS patients regardless of baseline low-density lipoprotein (LDL) levels. Specifically, high-intensity statins (eg,

Table 1
Pharmacologic treatment of acute coronary syndrome[9,11]

Drug	MOA	Dose	Comments (ADEs, Interactions, and so Forth)
Nitroglycerin	Increases coronary collateral flow via coronary artery dilation; decreases preload and reduces ventricular wall tension via peripheral venodilation	SL: 0.3–0.4 mg every 5 min (up to three tablets in 15-min period) IV: 5–10 mcg/min, titrate by 5 mcg/min every 5–10 min (maximum 400 mcg/min)	Adverse effects: headache, dizziness, hypotension Contraindicated with PDE-5 inhibitors Tachyphylaxis after 24–48 h of use Caution in right-sided (inferior) MI
Aspirin	Irreversible inhibition of platelet aggregation	PO: 162–325 mg (chewable formulation, non-enteric coated)	If aspirin/salicylate allergy, consider clopidogrel 300–600 mg
P2Y$_{12}$ Inhibitors			
Clopidogrel Ticagrelor Prasugrel Cangrelor	Prevents platelet aggregation by blocking P2Y$_{12}$ receptors on platelets (irreversible binding for clopidogrel and prasugrel)	PO: 300–600 mg load, then 75 mg daily PO: 180 mg load, then 90 mg twice daily (60 mg twice daily after 1 y of maintenance) PO: 60 mg load, then 10 mg daily IV: 30 mcg/kg bolus before PCI, then 4 mcg/kg/min infusion	Adverse effects: bleeding, dyspnea (ticagrelor), risk of bradyarrhythmias, and ventricular pauses (ticagrelor) Avoid if patient going for urgent CABG surgery Ticagrelor: avoid if history of ICH; concomitant maintenance aspirin dose should not exceed 100 mg Prasugrel: contraindicated if history of stroke/TIA; not recommended in patients ≥ 75 year old (increases the risk of fatal bleeding and ICH)
Anticoagulants			
Enoxaparin (LMWH) Unfractionated heparin	Factor-Xa and thrombin inhibitor	SQ: 1 mg/kg every 12 h (1 mg/kg every 24 h if CrCl < 30 mL/min) Consider initial 30 mg IV loading dose in select patients IV: 60 units/kg bolus (maximum 5000 units); initial infusion 12 units/kg/h (maximum 1000 units/h)	Adverse effects: bleeding Adjust bivalirudin infusion dose in severe renal dysfunction

(continued on next page)

Table 1
(continued)

Drug	MOA	Dose	Comments (ADEs, Interactions, and so Forth)
Bivalirudin	Direct thrombin inhibitor	IV: 0.1 mg/kg bolus, then 0.25 mg/kg/h infusion (for planned invasive strategy NSTE-ACS)	
GP IIb/IIIa Receptor Antagonists			
Eptifibatide	Prevents platelet aggregation by inhibiting binding of fibrinogen to GP IIb/IIIa receptors	IV: 180 mcg/kg bolus (maximum 22.6 mg), then 2 mcg/kg/min (maximum 15 mg/h) with second 180 mcg/kg bolus repeated 10 min after first	Not typically recommended for medical management without PCI Adverse effects: bleeding, thrombocytopenia, hypotension Reduce eptifibatide infusion 50% if CrCl < 50 mL/min; avoid in hemodialysis Reduce tirofiban infusion 50% if CrCl ≤ 60 mL/min
Tirofiban		IV: 25 mcg/kg bolus, then 0.15 mcg/kg/min	
Fibrinolytics			
Alteplase	Binds to fibrin and converts plasminogen to plasmin to initiate fibrinolysis	IV: 15 mg bolus, then 0.75 mg/kg infusion for 30 min (maximum 50 mg), then 0.5 mg/kg over next 60 min (maximum 35 mg); maximum dose 100 mg	Only used for STEMI Adverse effects: bleeding (including ICH), hypotension Different contraindications than those used for ischemic stroke indication Tenecteplase has higher fibrin specificity than alteplase or reteplase
Tenecteplase		IV push: < 60 kg: 30 mg 60–69 kg: 35 mg 70–79 kg: 40 mg 80–89 kg: 45 mg ≥ 90 kg: 50 mg	

Abbreviations: ADE, adverse drug event; CABG, cornary artery bypass graft; cAMP, cyclic adenosine monophosphate; GP, glycoprotein; ICH, intracranial hemorrhage; LMWH, low molecular weight heparin; MI, myocardial infarction; MOA, mechanism of action; PDE, phosphodiesterase; PO, by mouth; SL, sublingual; SQ, subcutaneous; STEMI, ST-elevation MI; TIA, transient ischemic attack

atorvastatin 40 to 80 mg or rosuvastatin 20 to 40 mg) improve mortality and reduce ischemic events in ACS patients.[13,14] Although not mentioned in current guidelines, utilization of a high-intensity statin "load" before PCI improves coronary perfusion and reduces inflammation and may be a consideration for patients in the ED.[15,16]

Acute Heart Failure

Patients with episodes of AHF may present to the ED for their index encounter or to address an abrupt worsening of their chronic heart failure symptoms. Prompt targeted therapy improves patient outcomes and limits hospital length of stay.[17] CS is the most critical form of AHF, though it only represents <5% of AHF cases.

Most of the patients presenting to the ED with AHF suffer from fluid overload and congestion to some degree and will likely benefit from administration of intravenous (IV) loop diuretics. The IV route is preferred over oral given variable absorption, especially during an AHF exacerbation.[18] For patients not on a loop diuretic at home, it is recommended to start with 20 to 40 mg IV furosemide (**Table 2**). Otherwise, patients should receive an IV dose 2 to 2.5 times their home daily dose.[19] Following adequate response to an IV loop diuretic, patients should be continued on an IV diuretic (either as a continuous infusion or as intermittent doses 2–3 times daily) until their fluid overload has resolved. Administration of an IV loop diuretic via an infusion is often preferred to scheduled bolus doses due to increased diuretic effect and safety, but this does not translate into reduced length of stay or mortality[20,21] Consider including a bolus whenever the infusion is uptitrated. In patients that do not respond adequately to an IV loop diuretic alone, the addition of an alternative diuretic, such as oral metolazone or IV chlorothiazide, may be considered in order to augment their diuresis. Alternatively, there is also a small subset of patients that may present with hypoperfusion and no signs of fluid overload who may benefit from small fluid boluses. These patients may be identified based on evaluation of a chest x-ray and bedside ultrasound.

Vasodilators (nitroglycerin and sodium nitroprusside) may be considered in patients with AHF who have pulmonary edema and a systolic blood pressure >110 mm Hg. This can help to both resolve congestion and offload the heart, though the GALACTIC trial found there was no difference between vasodilators and usual care in regard to 180-day mortality, AHF rehospitalizations, dyspnea, or N-terminal-proB-type natriuretic peptide (NT-proBNP) concentrations[24,25] Therefore, use of vasodilators may best be suited for treatment of sympathetic crashing acute pulmonary edema instead of heart failure.

Cardiogenic Shock

CS is a life-threatening form of AHF and carries a high rate of mortality. CS is typically defined as prolonged hypotension (systolic blood pressure <90 mm Hg) or vasopressor requirement to keep SBP >90 mm Hg in the absence of hypovolemia and

Table 2
Loop diuretic dose oral to intravenous conversion[22,23]

Medication	Oral (mg)	Intravenous (mg)
Furosemide	40–80	20–40
Torsemide	20	N/A
Bumetanide	1	1

with signs of hypoperfusion.[26] The most common form of CS is the "cold and wet" subset, in which patients are systemically vasoconstricted and fluid overloaded. As with less severe forms of AHF, patients with CS and fluid overload should receive aggressive IV diuresis with a loop diuretic. In addition to diuresis, inotropes and vaso-pressors are critical and potentially lifesaving interventions that can provide temporary support until more definitive interventions or until resolution of the underlying etiology of decompensation.[27] It is usually recommended to start with norepinephrine instead of an inotrope, as inotropes cause vasodilation and may worsen hypotension. When epinephrine was compared with norepinephrine for patients with CS, norepinephrine provided similar improvements in blood pressure and cardiac output with a lower inci-dence of refractory shock.[28] Following improvement in blood pressure, the addition of, or transition to, an inotrope can be considered. In the ED, dobutamine may be preferred to milrinone as dobutamine has a half-life of ~2 minutes, whereas milrinone has a half-life of ~2 hours. Milrinone is also renally eliminated and, as renal dysfunc-tion is a frequent complication of CS, the half-life of milrinone may be prolonged to > 20 hours, which can result in accumulation from rapid dose escalations. There does not seem to be a difference in meaningful outcomes between dobutamine and milri-none[29,30] **Table 3** outlines the medications used in CS.

Atrial Fibrillation

Introduction on rate versus rhythm control

There are generally two strategies for managing atrial fibrillation with rapid ventricular response (RVR): rhythm control or rate control. The former can be addressed with electrical cardioversion, medication therapy, and/or ablation, whereas the latter is generally treated with medications. The largest trial to compare these two approaches was published in 2002 by the AFFIRM investigators.[31] For long-term management of patients with atrial fibrillation, this study found no mortality difference between the rhythm and rate-control groups and noted advantages such as a lower risk of adverse effects with rate control, and a second study reached a similar conclusion.[32] The 2014 American Heart Association/American College of Cardiology/Heart Rhythm Society Guidelines recommend starting with rate control in most patients, relegating rhythm control to use in select populations, such as persistent symptoms, heart failure, or newly diagnosed patients who are at high risk for cardiovascular complications.[33]

The Canadian Association of Emergency Physicians periodically publishes an acute atrial fibrillation/flutter best practices checklist.[34] They state that initial assessment of ED patients with atrial fibrillation/flutter with RVR should evaluate whether the rapid rate is a primary arrhythmia or secondary to another medical cause. Second, is the pa-tient stable or unstable? Third, is cardioversion safe for the patient taking into account anticoagulation status and other factors?

Rate Control

If rate control is chosen, the first question that usually arises is whether to use a beta-blocker or calcium channel blocker (CCB). Metoprolol is the preferred beta-blocker. Diltiazem or verapamil is the preferred CCBs. If a patient is on an oral beta-blocker or non-dihydropyridine CCB at home, it is generally best to start with the IV equivalent of that same medication in the ED. If a patient is not on either at home, ED-based studies suggest a slightly higher success rate with choosing CCBs over beta-blockers[35–46] In fact, a 2021 meta-analysis of ED studies involving 1214 patients from nine randomized controlled trials and eight cohort studies confirmed this finding.[47]

Table 3
Pharmacologic treatment of cardiogenic shock

Drug	MOA	Route	Dose	Comments (ADEs, Interactions, and so Forth)
Furosemide	Inhibits reabsorption of sodium in ascending loop of Henle	IV/Oral	Initial: 20–40 mg 1–2 times daily or double home dose for AHF exacerbation IV infusion: starting at 10–20 mg/h; typical maximum 40 mg/h	Adverse effects: electrolyte disturbances, hypotension, metabolic alkalosis, ototoxicity (associated with high bolus doses, reversible), and myalgia (more common in bumetanide)
Torsemide		Oral	Initial: 10–20 mg daily	Presence of gut-wall edema will affect absorption
Bumetanide		IV/Oral	Initial: 0.5–1 mg 1–2 times daily or double home dose for AHF exacerbation IV infusion: starting at 0.5–1 mg/h; typical maximum 2 mg/h	
Metolazone	Inhibits reabsorption of sodium in distal tubules	Oral	Initial: 2.5–5 mg daily; maximum 20 mg daily	Adverse effects: electrolyte disturbances
Chlorothiazide		IV	Initial: 500–1000 mg daily as needed; maximum 2000 mg daily	Consider to give 30–60 min before loop diuretic bolus
Nitroglycerin	Forms nitric oxide in blood vessels which produces smooth muscle relaxation and vasodilation	IV	IV infusion: Starting at 10 mcg/min, up titrated by 10 mcg/min every 3–5 min as needed	Adverse effects: headache, dizziness, hypotension Venous (preload ↓) at lower doses Arterial (afterload ↓) at higher doses
Sodium nitroprusside		IV	IV infusion: starting at 0.1–0.2 mcg/kg/min, uptitrated by 0.1–0.2 mcg/kg/min every 5–10 min as needed	Adverse effects: cyanide/thiocyanate toxicity (increased risk if hepatic or renal impairment; prolonged use) Venous and arterial vasodilation
Epinephrine	Stimulates beta$_1$ > alpha$_1$ receptors to increase chronotropy, inotropy, and vasoconstriction	IV	IV infusion starting at 1–3 mcg/min or 0.01–0.05 mcg/kg/min (<5 mcg/min for inotropic effects)	Adverse effects: tachyarrhythmias, increased cardiac work

(continued on next page)

Table 3
(continued)

Drug	MOA	Route	Dose	Comments (ADEs, Interactions, and so Forth)
Norepinephrine	Stimulates $alpha_1$ > $beta_1$ receptors to increase vasoconstriction and blood pressure	IV	IV infusion starting at 3–5 mcg/min or 0.05 mcg/kg/min	Adverse effects: tachyarrhythmias
Dobutamine	Stimulates $beta_1$ receptors to increase chronotropy and inotropy	IV	IV infusion starting at 2–5 mcg/kg/min (maximum 20 mcg/kg/min)	Adverse effects: tachyarrhythmias Preferred in patients with hypotension (less vasodilatory than milrinone)
Milrinone	Phosphodiesterase-3 inhibitor which increases cAMP to increase chronotropy and inotropy	IV	IV infusion starting at 0.1–2 mcg/kg/min (maximum 0.75 mcg/kg/min)	Adverse effects: tachyarrhythmias Preferred in patients with pulmonary hypertension or right heart failure (reducing pulmonary vascular resistance)

Emergency clinicians should also think beyond the ED and consider other medical conditions a patient may have when choosing an initial rate control agent. For example, heart failure with reduced ejection fraction or ischemic heart disease is better managed with beta-blockers. In patients with concomitant hypertension who may benefit from additional blood pressure lowering, CCBs may be a more ideal option for rate control.

Dosing for metoprolol is generally 2.5 to 5 mg IV every 15 minutes up to 3 doses.[34] Historically, diltiazem is dosed based on weight at 0.25 mg/kg initially, repeated every 15 minutes at 0.35 mg/kg up to three doses. However, one ED group compared a fixed 10 mg dose to weight-based dosing and found similar success between the two strategies.[48] A second study also found no difference in therapeutic response, though those receiving weight-based dosing did reach an heart rate (HR) < 100 bpm more often.[49] The investigators proposed that ideal body weight be used when using weight-based dosing. Irrespective of which dosing method is chosen, most patients require about 30 mg.[50] Consider using the 10 mg strategy in patients with borderline initial blood pressures, older adults, and those anticipated to drop their blood pressure.

Some studies suggest CCBs cause more hypotension than beta-blockers. Calcium supplementation may prevent further decreases in blood pressure while not affecting the ability of the treatment to effectively lower heart rate. Most of the data are with verapamil and the numbers are small (**Table 4**). All of the studies used weight-based dosing of the CCB.

Magnesium

Over the years, IV magnesium has been studied for the treatment of rapid AF both as a primary therapy and as an adjunct. In fact, two meta-analyses from 2007[60,61] concluded that magnesium is safe and effective in controlling ventricular rate in rapid AF compared with placebo, the latter in patients also receiving digoxin. A closer look at the meta-analyses reveals that the positive rate-control effect for magnesium seems to be driven by the placebo-controlled trials.[62] Of the 11 studies cited in the meta-analyses, only five reported rate-control data in ED-related settings.[63–67] Since the meta-analysis was concluded, two additional studies were published.[68,69]

The LOMAGHI study found 4.5 gm of IV magnesium (when combined with an atrioventricular [AV] nodal blocking agent) achieved the heart rate outcome better than placebo (64.2% vs 43.6% at 4 hours; 97.9% vs 83.3% at 24 hours).[69] Greater decreases in heart rate throughout the 24-h study period were achieved with the addition of magnesium. This is important because it may not be immediately evident during an ED stay if magnesium is helping, especially when using digoxin which takes longer to work (peak effects may take up to 6 hours). In addition, the most common AV nodal blocking agent in the study was digoxin and this is not reflective of general practice in the Unite States.

Based on the available data, the magnesium dose should be 2 to 4 gm IV infused over 15 to 30 minutes. The primary adverse effects of IV magnesium are flushing and hypotension which are rate related, as is the efficacy. Although not mentioned in the guidelines, IV magnesium may be an effective adjunctive agent for achieving rate control in the ED.

Special situations

If one rate-control agent is not effective after appropriate dosing, the question often arises as to whether it is safe to switch to another AV nodal blocking agent. Historically, the combination of two different parenteral AV nodal blockers was avoided due to

Table 4
Effect of calcium supplementation on blood pressure in patient with rapid atrial arrhythmias

Citation	Study Design	N	Drug	Calcium Form/Dose	Results
Weiss 1983[51]	Prospective	13	Verapamil	Calcium gluconate 1 gm	SBP ↑ 5 mm Hg
Roguin 1984[52]	Case series	2	Verapamil	Calcium gluconate (pediatrics)	No hypotension
Haft 1986[53]	Sequential study of two treatment protocols	50	Verapamil	Calcium chloride 1 gm	SBP ↑ 2 mm Hg
Salerno 1987[54]	Sequential study of two treatment protocols	5	Verapamil	Calcium gluconate 1 gm	SBP ↓ 12 mm Hg
Stringer 1988[55]	Case report	1	Verapamil	Calcium chloride 1 gm	No hypotension
Barnett 1990[56]	Prospective report of protocol	19	Verapamil	Calcium chloride 1 gm or calcium gluconate 1 gm	SBP ↑ 4 mm Hg
Kuhn 1992[57]	Retrospective	18	Verapamil	Calcium chloride 1 gm or calcium gluconate 3 gm	No hypotension
Miyagawa 1993[58]	Sequential study of two treatment protocols	7	Verapamil	Calcium gluconate 3.75 mg/kg	SBP: no change
Kolkebeck 2004[59]	Prospective, randomized, double-blind, placebo-controlled	34	Diltiazem	Calcium chloride 0.333 gm	SBP ↓ 8 mm Hg (placebo had SBP ↓ 14 mm Hg)

Abbreviation: SBP, systolic blood pressure.

the perceived risk, and anecdotal cases of bradycardia, and/or heart block. One hundred thirty-six patients who received the combination of IV beta-blocker and IV CCB within 4 hours of each other were evaluated.[70] Bradycardia developed in 4% of cases (one patient required intervention) and 9% developed hypotension with systolic blood pressures as low as 72 mm Hg. So, combination therapy is not benign but it seems to rarely lead to heart block; caution is advised. Consider separating the agents by as much time as is clinically feasible and using the fixed-dose strategy with diltiazem if switching from metoprolol.

All of the AV nodal blocking agents (metoprolol, diltiazem, verapamil) possess negative inotropic effects. As such, there is concern about their use in heart failure patients with reduced ejection fraction, particularly the CCBs. Available data suggest their use does not seem to be associated with risk for hypotension or other adverse events.[71,44] In a patient with severely reduced ejection fraction or acute decompensated heart failure, consider an alternative such as digoxin.

Rhythm control

Several options exist for pharmacologic rhythm control, but the data in ED patients largely support procainamide.[72,73,34] Amiodarone has a slow onset and limited efficacy. A reasonably simplified dosing strategy originated from the Ottawa Aggressive Protocol and was subsequently validated in over 1000 ED patients with recent-onset atrial fibrillation and flutter.[72,73] Procainamide 15 mg/kg is infused over 60 minutes. The Canadian guidelines recommend a max of 1500 mg, though we prefer to cap at 1000 mg. Procainamide should be avoided if the systolic blood pressure is less than 100 mm Hg or the QTc interval is greater than 500 msec. Although the medication is infusing, close monitoring is required and it should be stopped if the blood pressure drops or the QRS complex on ECG (QRS) interval lengthens significantly (eg, >30%). Other rhythm control options include flecainide, ibutilide, and propafenone.

Supraventricular Tachycardia

For undifferentiated SVT not relieved by Valsalva maneuvers in the hemodynamically stable patient, IV adenosine or IV nondihydropyridine CCBs (verapamil or diltiazem) are recommended, with adenosine being first-line due to its rapid onset and short half-life of seconds as well as safety profile (**Table 5**). However, the rapidity with which

Table 5
Pharmacologic treatment of supraventricular tachycardia

Drug	MOA	Route	Dose	Comments
Adenosine	Slows conduction through AV node	IV	Rapid IV bolus 6 mg, followed by 12 mg if ineffective	Adverse effects: transient AV block, flushing, headache, dizziness Must be given quickly given short half-life <10 s
Diltiazem	Inhibits the inflow of calcium ions during depolarization	IV	0.25 mg/kg (or 10 mg), followed by 0.35 mg/kg (or 20 mg) if needed	May cause hypotension if given by rapid IV push
Verapamil	preventing contraction	IV	5–10 mg, repeat if needed	

adenosine is inactivated may also lead to higher rates of recurrence of SVT compared with CCBs. Overall, the efficacy of adenosine and CCBs are similar at 85% to 90% and 90% to 98%, respectively.[74–77] Adenosine inhibits conduction at the AV node and increases the refractory period.[78] The dosing of adenosine is 6 mg with a subsequent dose of 12 mg if needed. Higher doses may be required if the patient recently consumed caffeine or theophylline as these have chemical structures similar to adenine and act as competitive inhibitors at the adenosine receptors.[79] Conversely, if a central line is used for administration, if the patient is on dipyridamole or carbamazepine, or if the patient is a cardiac transplant recipient, then the dose may be halved. Adenosine should be given by rapid IV bolus into a proximal vein followed immediately by a 20 mL saline flush. If adenosine is not effective then diltiazem or verapamil should be trialed. One concern with CCBs is the occurrence of hypotension post-administration.[80] Infusing the CCB over 10 minutes rather than IV bolus or pretreatment with calcium gluconate has been shown to decrease the occurrence of hypotension.[81] Synchronized cardioversion is recommended for hemodynamically unstable SVT.

Torsades de Pointes

TdP is a type of polymorphic ventricular tachycardia associated with QTc prolongation that is either congenital or acquired. There is an increased risk of TdP whenever the QTc exceeds 500 mg, or if drug induced when the QTc increases by > 60 msec following drug administration. Medications that are often incited as potentially provoking TdP are class Ia (sotalol, dofetilide—risk lower with sotalol) and III (amiodarone, dronedarone) antiarrhythmics, tricyclic antidepressants, typical and atypical antipsychotics, and fluoroquinolone antibiotics being at the top of the list.[82,83] The mechanism of these medications all have in common is their blockade of rectified potassium current (Ikr), a potassium channel that impacts repolarization of the cardiac action potential. When this is blocked there is prolongation of ventricular repolarization, thereby increasing this risk of early after depolarizations.[84] Drug-related QTc prolongation can be exacerbated by certain factors such as electrolyte abnormalities (hypokalemia, hypocalcemia, hypomagnesemia), older age, female gender, and heart disease.[85]

Appropriate management of TdP depends on the hemodynamic stability of the patient (**Table 6**). If the patient is hypotensive or in VF, then immediate cardioversion or defibrillation should be performed. If the patient is hemodynamically stable, magnesium sulfate is the treatment of choice due to its stabilizing effect on the cardiac

Table 6
Pharmacologic treatment of torsades de pointes

Drug	MOA	Route	Dose	Comments
Magnesium sulfate	Stabilizes cardiac myocardium	IV	2 g over 10 min, repeat if needed	May cause flushing and hypotension
Isoproterenol	Beta 1 receptor agonist	IV	2–10 mcg/min continuous infusion titrated to goal heart rate 90–100 bpm	Avoid if patient has congenital long-QT syndrome
Lidocaine	Blocks voltage gated sodium channels	IV	1–1.5 mg/kg (max 100 mg), followed by 1 mg/min continuous infusion	Avoid if patient has severe sinus node dysfunction or advanced AV block

myocardium. If multiple doses of magnesium sulfate are ineffective to restore a perfusing rhythm and the patient does not have a history of congenital prolonged QTc, isoproterenol may be considered to speed the heart rate, shorten the QTc, and lessen the likelihood of R-on-T. Isoproterenol is a nonselective beta agonist and is most effective if the patient is bradycardic before initiating therapy.[86] There may be logistical issues surrounding isoproterenol in that it is expensive and often not readily available on patient care floors, which can delay its acquisition and administration. Antiarrhythmic drugs that prolong ventricular repolarization should be avoided (class Ia, Ic, and III).[87] In refractory cases, there is limited evidence that class Ib agents, specifically lidocaine, may successfully terminate TdP, however, these data are limited to dog and rabbit models as well as a few human case reports.[88–91]

Ventricular Fibrillation/Pulseless Ventricular Tachycardia

VF and pulseless ventricular tachycardia (pVT) are two types of commonly seen rhythms in cardiac arrest and are considered "shockable," so attempts at defibrillation should be made in addition to pharmacologic intervention.[92] The management of VF and pVT should always begin with initiation of high-quality CPR and attempts at defibrillation should be made as soon as possible.[93] The advanced cardiovascular life support (ACLS) algorithms continue to emphasize early administration of epinephrine, as it has been shown to significantly improve return of spontaneous circulation (ROSC) and survival to hospital discharge.[94,95] However, it has not demonstrated a benefit in neurologic outcome, with a large randomized trial in 2018 showing that patients receiving epinephrine in out-of-hospital cardiac arrest had more severe neurologic impairment at discharge.[96] Epinephrine stimulates both beta- and alpha-adrenergic receptors, resulting in increased contractility and heart rate and vasoconstriction of vascular smooth muscle, respectively. Epinephrine should be administered every 3 to 5 minutes in addition to continuation of CPR and defibrillation attempts. If ROSC is still not obtained, the ACLS guidelines recommend administration of either amiodarone or lidocaine. Amiodarone blocks potassium channels to prolong repolarization, slow sinus rate, and increase AV node refractoriness, while also possessing beta-blockade and effects on sodium and calcium channels. However, due to delayed onset as an antiarrhythmic, its predominant effects in the immediate period are primarily electrophysiologic via beta-adrenergic blockade. Lidocaine blocks sodium channels to slow conduction and suppress myocardial automaticity. It is important to note that these antiarrhythmic agents have been proven to facilitate termination of VF/pVT and improve survival to hospital admission, but have not yet demonstrated any long-term benefit in cardiac arrest.[97–99] The current guidelines do not favor one antiarrhythmic agent over the other in this situation. Epinephrine, amiodarone, and lidocaine can all be administered either IV or intraosseously (IO) during VF/pVT; however, the most recent ACLS guidelines now prefer IV over IO if feasible.[100] In patients with refractory VF ($\geq$3 defibrillation attempts, 3 mg IV epinephrine total, and 300 mg IV amiodarone), two studies have demonstrated potentially improved outcomes with esmolol when given as a bolus followed by an infusion.[101,102] Both studies were small, but they both seemed to suggest improved rates of sustained ROSC and neurologic function. In cardiac arrest, excessive amounts of endogenous and exogenous catecholamines (namely epinephrine) may increase myocardial oxygen demand and lower the ventricular fibrillation threshold via beta$_1$ stimulation, as esmolol is an ultrashort-acting beta$_1$ selective adrenergic antagonist it may help to attenuate these issues. **Table 7** describes the medication management of VF and pVT.

Table 7
Pharmacologic treatment of ventricular fibrillation and VT

Drug	MOA	Route	Dose	Comments (ADEs, Interactions, and so Forth)
Amiodarone	Class Ia: sodium channel blocker Class II: beta-blocker Class III: potassium channel blocker Class IV: calcium channel blocker	IV	IV bolus 150 mg over 10 min, followed by 1 mg/min for 6 h then 0.5 mg/min over 18 h Additional boluses of 150 mg may be given as needed VF/pVT: IV 300 mg push, may repeat with 150 mg	Adverse effects: pulmonary toxicity, thyroid toxicity, bradycardia, AV block, hepatotoxicity (acute hepatic failure; chronic hepatic fibrosis) Rapid infusion may lead to hypotension and pulseless arrhythmias Full antiarrhythmic effect not seen for days–weeks (half-life ∼ 50 d)
Epinephrine	Increases contractility and heart rate, vasoconstricts vascular smooth muscle	IV	VF/pVT: IV 1 mg push every 3–5 min	Adverse effects: tachyarrhythmias, increased cardiac work
Esmolol	Class II: beta-blocker	IV	IV bolus 500 mcg/kg, followed by an IV infusion at 50–100 mcg/kg/min	Adverse effects: bradycardia, hypotension Easily titratable due to half-life of 9 min Selective for beta-1 receptors
Lidocaine	Class Ib: sodium channel blocker	IV	IV bolus 1–1.5 mg/kg (usually 100 mg), followed by 0.5–0.75 mg/kg every 5–10 min as needed, followed by an infusion starting at 1 mg/min	Adverse effects: headache, confusion, tremors, seizures May be preferred if the arrhythmia is secondary to an ischemic event/infarction Consider lidocaine levels for prolonged infusions or at a high rate, if there are signs/symptoms of toxicity, or patients have renal or hepatic impairment
Procainamide	Class Ia: sodium channel blocker	IV	Slow IV bolus of 10–17 mg/kg at a rate of 20–50 mg/min continued until the arrhythmia is controlled, hypotension occurs, QRS widens by 50%, or a maximum of 17 mg/kg Followed by an infusion at 1–4 mg/min	Adverse effects: drug-induced lupus, agranulocytosis, positive ANA, confusion Consider procainamide (4–10 mcg/mL) or NAPA level (15–25 mcg/mL) with prolonged infusion
Sotalol	Class II: beta-blocker Class III: Potassium channel blocker	IV	IV bolus 1.5 mg/kg (or 100 mg) over 5 min	Adverse effects: QTc prolongation

Stable Ventricular Tachycardia

Stable ventricular tachycardia (HR > 120–130 bpm) is a wide complex (QRS >120 msec) arrhythmia that is less frequently encountered in the ED. In order to be considered stable, patients must not have hypotension, altered mental status, chest pain, or heart failure. If any of these are present but the patient has a pulse, then they should receive immediate synchronized cardioversion. In addition, if patients become clinically unstable during any of the pharmacologic therapies, synchronized cardioversion is recommended and is more effective than any antiarrhythmic. If there is concern for electrical storm causing a wide complex tachycardia (WCT), esmolol should be considered. For patients with a monomorphic regular WCT, adenosine may be considered as it can help terminate SVT with aberrancy or help diagnose other atrial arrhythmias as it will slow conduction through the AV node. If adenosine is ineffective or not administered, IV antiarrhythmics are typically the next step. The 2020 AHA ACLS guidelines provide a 2b (weak, benefit ≥ risk) recommendation based on moderate quality evidence stating that IV amiodarone, procainamide, or sotalol may be considered for WCT.[92] They purposefully chose to not recommend lidocaine for undifferentiated WCT as it is not effective for SVT and less effective than the other medications for ventricular tachycardia (VT). There are numerous heterogeneous small studies that evaluate the various antiarrhythmics, with mixed findings. The PROCA-MIO study is likely one of the most impactful.[103] They randomized 62 patients with stable monomorphic WCT to either IV procainamide (*n* = 33) or IV amiodarone (*n* = 29) given via a bolus and infusion. After 40 minutes following the bolus, significantly more patients in the procainamide group had resolution of their WCT than those in the amiodarone group (67% vs 38%). In addition, patients who received procainamide had significantly fewer major cardiac events during the study period (3% vs 12%). Based on this study and others where procainamide was also superior to lidocaine and amiodarone, it may be reasonable to consider procainamide as the first-line antiarrhythmic for stable WCT, unless other factors are present to suggest otherwise.[104–106] Following successful chemical cardioversion, a continuous infusion of the successful agent is not required but may be continued based on expert opinion and suspected etiology.

SUMMARY

Pharmacologic therapy is a vital component in the management of many cardiovascular emergencies. Knowledge of the mechanisms of action is helpful in understanding which treatment option may be best for an individual patient. Choosing the appropriate dose and route, while taking into account clinically significant adverse effects and drug interactions, is also important. Most cardiovascular emergency drug therapy is supported by national and international guidelines, though there are some nuanced approaches such as using magnesium in atrial fibrillation with RVR. Pharmacologic interventions are often complementary to non-pharmacologic ones such as PCI or electrical cardioversion/defibrillation; optimal patient outcomes are achieved with timely initiation of both.

CLINICS CARE POINTS

- Emergency Department management of myocardial infarction prior to cardiac catheterizaion laboratory intervnetion generally includes aspirin, heparin or low molecular weight heparin, a statin, and a P2Y12 inhibitor.

- In atrial fibrillation patients needing acute rate control, begin with the IV formulation of the home regimen (eg, beta blocker or calcium channel blocker). If the patient is not on any home medications, calcium channel blockers may offer a small advantage over beta blockers for rate control in the Emergency Department.
- When using adenosine, alternative administration techniques such as mixing it with the flush fluid, are effective.

DISCLOSURE

The authors have nothing to disclose.

REFERENCES

1. Meyers HP, Bracey A, Lee D, et al. Comparison of the ST-Elevation Myocardial Infarction (STEMI) vs. NSTEMI and Occlusion MI (OMI) vs. NOMI Paradigms of Acute MI. J Emerg Med 2021;60:273–84.
2. Meine TJ, Roe MT, Chen AY, et al. Association of intravenous morphine use and outcomes in acute coronary syndromes: results from the CRUSADE Quality Improvement Initiative. Am Heart J 2005;149:1043–9.
3. Kubica J, Adamski P, Ostrowska M, et al. Morphine delays and attenuates ticagrelor exposure and action in patients with myocardial infarction: the randomized, double-blind, placebo-controlled IMPRESSION trial. Eur Heart J 2016; 37:245–52.
4. Hobl E-L, Stimpfl T, Ebner J, et al. Morphine decreases clopidogrel concentrations and effects: a randomized, double-blind, placebo-controlled trial. J Am Coll Cardiol 2014;63:630–5.
5. Parodi G, Valenti R, Bellandi B, et al. Comparison of prasugrel and ticagrelor loading doses in ST-segment elevation myocardial infarction patients: RAPID (Rapid Activity of Platelet Inhibitor Drugs) primary PCI study. J Am Coll Cardiol 2013;61:1601–6.
6. Gibson CM, Pride YB, Aylward PE, et al. Association of non-steroidal anti-inflammatory drugs with outcomes in patients with ST-segment elevation myocardial infarction treated with fibrinolytic therapy: an ExTRACT-TIMI 25 analysis. J Thromb Thrombolysis 2009;27:11–7.
7. Gislason GH, Jacobsen S, Rasmussen JN, et al. Risk of death or reinfarction associated with the use of selective cyclooxygenase-2 inhibitors and nonselective nonsteroidal antiinflammatory drugs after acute myocardial infarction. Circulation 2006;113:2906–13.
8. Ibanez B, James S, Agewall S, et al. 2017 ESC Guidelines for the management of acute myocardial infarction in patients presenting with ST-segment elevation: The Task Force for the management of acute myocardial infarction in patients presenting with ST-segment elevation of the European Society of Cardiology (ESC). Eur Heart J 2018;39:119–77.
9. O'Gara PT, Kushner FG, Ascheim DD, et al. 2013 ACCF/AHA guideline for the management of ST-elevation myocardial infarction: a report of the American College of Cardiology Foundation/American Heart Association Task Force on Practice Guidelines. Circulation 2013;127:e362–425.
10. Levine GN, Bates ER, Bittl JA, et al. 2016 ACC/AHA Guideline Focused Update on Duration of Dual Antiplatelet Therapy in Patients With Coronary Artery Disease: A Report of the American College of Cardiology/American Heart Association Task Force on Clinical Practice Guidelines: An Update of the 2011 ACCF/

AHA/SCAI Guideline for Percutaneous Coronary Intervention, 2011 ACCF/AHA Guideline for Coronary Artery Bypass Graft Surgery, 2012 ACC/AHA/ACP/AATS/PCNA/SCAI/STS Guideline for the Diagnosis and Management of Patients With Stable Ischemic Heart Disease, 2013 ACCF/AHA Guideline for the Management of ST-Elevation Myocardial Infarction, 2014 AHA/ACC Guideline for the Management of Patients With Non-ST-Elevation Acute Coronary Syndromes, and 2014 ACC/AHA Guideline on Perioperative Cardiovascular Evaluation and Management of Patients Undergoing Noncardiac Surgery. Circulation 2016; 134:e123–55.

11. Amsterdam EA, Wenger NK, Brindis RG, et al. 2014 AHA/ACC guideline for the management of patients with non-ST-elevation acute coronary syndromes: a report of the American college of cardiology/American heart association task force on practice guidelines. J Am Coll Cardiol 2014;64:e139–228.

12. Oler A, Whooley MA, Oler J, et al. Adding heparin to aspirin reduces the incidence of myocardial infarction and death in patients with unstable angina. a meta-analysis. JAMA 1996;276:811–5.

13. Cannon CP, Braunwald E, McCabe CH, et al. Intensive versus moderate lipid lowering with statins after acute coronary syndromes. N Engl J Med 2004; 350:1495–504.

14. Schwartz GG, Olsson AG, Ezekowitz MD, et al. Effects of atorvastatin on early recurrent ischemic events in acute coronary syndromes: the MIRACL study: a randomized controlled trial. JAMA 2001;285:1711–8.

15. Kim J-S, Kim J, Choi D, et al. Efficacy of high-dose atorvastatin loading before primary percutaneous coronary intervention in ST-segment elevation myocardial infarction: the STATIN STEMI trial. JACC Cardiovasc Interv 2010;3:332–9.

16. Liu H-L, Yang Y, Yang S-L, et al. Administration of a loading dose of atorvastatin before percutaneous coronary intervention prevents inflammation and reduces myocardial injury in STEMI patients: a randomized clinical study. Clin Ther 2013;35:261–72.

17. Mebazaa A, Tolppanen H, Mueller C, et al. Acute heart failure and cardiogenic shock: a multidisciplinary practical guidance. Intensive Care Med 2016;42: 147–63.

18. Sica DA. Pharmacotherapy in congestive heart failure: drug absorption in the management of congestive heart failure: loop diuretics. Congest Heart Fail 2003;9:287–92.

19. Felker GM, Lee KL, Bull DA, et al. Diuretic strategies in patients with acute decompensated heart failure. N Engl J Med 2011;364:797–805.

20. Salvador DRK, Rey NR, Ramos GC, et al. Continuous infusion versus bolus injection of loop diuretics in congestive heart failure. Cochrane Database Syst Rev 2004;2005(3):CD003178.

21. Ng KT, Yap JLL. Continuous infusion vs. intermittent bolus injection of furosemide in acute decompensated heart failure: systematic review and meta-analysis of randomised controlled trials. Anaesthesia 2018;73:238–47.

22. Brisco-Bacik MA, Ter Maaten JM, Houser SR, et al. Outcomes associated with a strategy of adjuvant metolazone or high-dose loop diuretics in acute decompensated heart failure: a propensity analysis. J Am Heart Assoc 2018;7:e009149.

23. Catlin JR, Adams CB, Louie DJ, et al. Aggressive versus conservative initial diuretic dosing in the emergency department for acute decompensated heart failure. Ann Pharmacother 2018;52:26–31.

24. Kozhuharov N, Goudev A, Flores D, et al. Effect of a strategy of comprehensive vasodilation vs usual care on mortality and heart failure rehospitalization among

patients with acute heart failure: the galactic randomized clinical trial. JAMA 2019;322:2292–302.

25. WRITING COMMITTEE MEMBERS, Yancy CW, Jessup M, et al. 2013 ACCF/AHA guideline for the management of heart failure: a report of the American College of Cardiology Foundation/American Heart Association Task Force on practice guidelines. Circulation 2013;128:e240–327.

26. Vahdatpour C, Collins D, Goldberg S. Cardiogenic Shock. J Am Heart Assoc 2019;8:e011991.

27. Yancy CW, Jessup M, Bozkurt B, et al. 2013 ACCF/AHA guideline for the management of heart failure: a report of the American College of Cardiology Foundation/American Heart Association Task Force on Practice Guidelines. J Am Coll Cardiol 2013;62:e147–239.

28. Levy B, Clere-Jehl R, Legras A, et al. Epinephrine versus norepinephrine for cardiogenic shock after acute myocardial infarction. J Am Coll Cardiol 2018; 72:173–82.

29. Mathew R, Di Santo P, Jung RG, et al. Milrinone as compared with dobutamine in the treatment of cardiogenic shock. N Engl J Med 2021;385:516–25.

30. Kelly J, Cheng J, Malloy R, et al. Comparison of Positive Inotropic Agents in the Management of Acute Decompensated Heart Failure. J Cardiovasc Pharmacol 2020;75:455–9.

31. Wyse DG, Waldo AL, DiMarco JP, et al. A comparison of rate control and rhythm control in patients with atrial fibrillation. N Engl J Med 2002;347:1825–33.

32. Van Gelder IC, Hagens VE, Bosker HA, et al. A comparison of rate control and rhythm control in patients with recurrent persistent atrial fibrillation. N Engl J Med 2002;347:1834–40.

33. January CT, Wann LS, Alpert JS, et al. 2014 AHA/ACC/HRS guideline for the management of patients with atrial fibrillation: a report of the American College of Cardiology/American Heart Association Task Force on Practice Guidelines and the Heart Rhythm Society. J Am Coll Cardiol 2014;64:e1–76.

34. Stiell IG, de Wit K, Scheuermeyer FX, et al. 2021 CAEP acute atrial fibrillation/flutter best practices checklist. CJEM 2021;23:604–10.

35. Demircan C, Cikriklar HI, Engindeniz Z, et al. Comparison of the effectiveness of intravenous diltiazem and metoprolol in the management of rapid ventricular rate in atrial fibrillation. Emerg Med J 2005;22:411–4.

36. Vinson DR, Hoehn T, Graber DJ, et al. Managing emergency department patients with recent-onset atrial fibrillation. J Emerg Med 2012;42:139–48.

37. Scheuermeyer FX, Grafstein E, Stenstrom R, et al. Safety and efficiency of calcium channel blockers versus beta-blockers for rate control in patients with atrial fibrillation and no acute underlying medical illness. Acad Emerg Med 2013;20:222–30.

38. Hassan S, Slim AM, Kamalakannan D, et al. Conversion of atrial fibrillation to sinus rhythm during treatment with intravenous esmolol or diltiazem: a prospective, randomized comparison. J Cardiovasc Pharmacol Ther 2007;12:227–31.

39. Martindale JL, deSouza IS, Silverberg M, et al. β-Blockers versus calcium channel blockers for acute rate control of atrial fibrillation with rapid ventricular response: a systematic review. Eur J Emerg Med 2015;22:150–4.

40. Fromm C, Suau SJ, Cohen V, et al. Diltiazem vs. metoprolol in the management of atrial fibrillation or flutter with rapid ventricular rate in the emergency department. J Emerg Med 2015;49:175–82.

41. McGrath P, Kersten B, Chilbert MR, et al. Evaluation of metoprolol versus diltiazem for rate control of atrial fibrillation in the emergency department. Am J Emerg Med 2021;46:585–90.

42. Nuñez Cruz S, DeMott JM, Peksa GD, et al. Evaluation of the blood pressure effects of diltiazem versus metoprolol in the acute treatment of atrial fibrillation with rapid ventricular rate. Am J Emerg Med 2021;46:329–34.

43. Hargrove KL, Robinson EE, Lusk KA, et al. Comparison of sustained rate control in atrial fibrillation with rapid ventricular rate: Metoprolol vs. Diltiazem. Am J Emerg Med 2021;40:15–9.

44. Hirschy R, Ackerbauer KA, Peksa GD, et al. Metoprolol vs. diltiazem in the acute management of atrial fibrillation in patients with heart failure with reduced ejection fraction. Am J Emerg Med 2019;37:80–4.

45. Nicholson J, Czosnowski Q, Flack T, et al. Hemodynamic comparison of intravenous push diltiazem versus metoprolol for atrial fibrillation rate control. Am J Emerg Med 2020;38:1879–83.

46. Hines MC, Reed BN, Ivaturi V, et al. Diltiazem versus metoprolol for rate control in atrial fibrillation with rapid ventricular response in the emergency department. Am J Health Syst Pharm 2016;73:2068–76.

47. Lan Q, Wu F, Han B, et al. Intravenous diltiazem versus metoprolol for atrial fibrillation with rapid ventricular rate: A meta-analysis. Am J Emerg Med 2021;51:248–56.

48. Ross AL, O'Sullivan DM, Drescher MJ, et al. Comparison of weight-based dose vs. standard dose diltiazem in patients with atrial fibrillation presenting to the emergency department. J Emerg Med 2016;51:440–6.

49. Ward SM, Radke J, Calhoun C, et al. Weight-based versus non-weight-based diltiazem dosing in the setting of atrial fibrillation with rapid ventricular response. Am J Emerg Med 2020;38:2271–6.

50. Zimmerman DE, Jachim L, Iaria A, et al. The effect of body weight on intravenous diltiazem in patients with atrial fibrillation with rapid ventricular response. J Clin Pharm Ther 2018;43:855–9.

51. Weiss AT, Lewis BS, Halon DA, et al. The use of calcium with verapamil in the management of supraventricular tachyarrhythmias. Int J Cardiol 1983;4:275–84.

52. Roguin N, Shapir Y, Blazer S, et al. The use of calcium gluconate prior to verapamil in infants with paroxysmal supraventricular tachycardia. Clin Cardiol 1984;7:613–6.

53. Haft JI, Habbab MA. Treatment of atrial arrhythmias. Effectiveness of verapamil when preceded by calcium infusion. Arch Intern Med 1986;146:1085–9.

54. Salerno DM, Anderson B, Sharkey PJ, et al. Intravenous verapamil for treatment of multifocal atrial tachycardia with and without calcium pretreatment. Ann Intern Med 1987;107:623–8.

55. Stringer KA, Hicks P, Royal SH, et al. Verapamil preceded by calcium in supraventricular tachycardia. Drug Intell Clin Pharm 1988;22:575–6.

56. Barnett JC, Touchon RC. Short-term control of supraventricular tachycardia with verapamil infusion and calcium pretreatment. Chest 1990;97:1106–9.

57. Kuhn M, Schriger DL. Low-dose calcium pretreatment to prevent verapamil-induced hypotension. Am Heart J 1992;124:231–2.

58. Miyagawa K, Dohi Y, Ogihara M, et al. Administration of intravenous calcium before verapamil to prevent hypotension in elderly patients with paroxysmal supraventricular tachycardia. J Cardiovasc Pharmacol 1993;22:273–9.

59. Kolkebeck T, Abbrescia K, Pfaff J, et al. Calcium chloride before i.v. diltiazem in the management of atrial fibrillation. J Emerg Med 2004;26:395–400.

60. Ho KM, Sheridan DJ, Paterson T. Use of intravenous magnesium to treat acute onset atrial fibrillation: a meta-analysis. Heart 2007;93:1433–40.
61. Onalan O, Crystal E, Daoulah A, et al. Meta-analysis of magnesium therapy for the acute management of rapid atrial fibrillation. Am J Cardiol 2007;99:1726–32.
62. Nair GM, Morillo CA. Magnesium in the acute management of atrial fibrillation: noise or music? Pol Arch Med Wewn 2007;117:446–7.
63. Chiladakis JA, Stathopoulos C, Davlouros P, et al. Intravenous magnesium sulfate versus diltiazem in paroxysmal atrial fibrillation. Int J Cardiol 2001;79: 287–91.
64. Davey MJ, Teubner D. A randomized controlled trial of magnesium sulfate, in addition to usual care, for rate control in atrial fibrillation. Ann Emerg Med 2005;45:347–53.
65. Joshi PP, Deshmukh PK, Salkar RG. Efficacy of intravenous magnesium sulphate in supraventricular tachyarrhythmias. J Assoc Physicians India 1995;43: 529–31.
66. Hays JV, Gilman JK, Rubal BJ. Effect of magnesium sulfate on ventricular rate control in atrial fibrillation. Ann Emerg Med 1994;24:61–4.
67. Gullestad L, Birkeland K, Mølstad P, et al. The effect of magnesium versus verapamil on supraventricular arrhythmias. Clin Cardiol 1993;16:429–34.
68. Chu K, Evans R, Emerson G, et al. Magnesium sulfate versus placebo for paroxysmal atrial fibrillation: a randomized clinical trial. Acad Emerg Med 2009;16: 295–300.
69. Bouida W, Beltaief K, Msolli MA, et al. Low-dose magnesium sulfate versus high dose in the early management of rapid atrial fibrillation: randomized controlled double-blind study (LOMAGHI study). Acad Emerg Med 2019;26:183–91.
70. Alowais SA, Hayes BD, Wilcox SR, et al. Heart rate outcomes with concomitant parenteral calcium channel blockers and beta blockers in rapid atrial fibrillation or flutter. Am J Emerg Med 2021;44:407–10.
71. Jandali MB. Safety of intravenous diltiazem in reduced ejection fraction heart failure with rapid atrial fibrillation. Clin Drug Investig 2018;38:503–8.
72. Stiell IG, Clement CM, Perry JJ, et al. Association of the Ottawa Aggressive Protocol with rapid discharge of emergency department patients with recent-onset atrial fibrillation or flutter. CJEM 2010;12:181–91.
73. Stiell IG, Clement CM, Rowe BH, et al. Outcomes for emergency department patients with recent-onset atrial fibrillation and flutter treated in Canadian hospitals. Ann Emerg Med 2017;69:562–71.e2.
74. Lim SH, Anantharaman V, Teo WS, et al. Slow infusion of calcium channel blockers compared with intravenous adenosine in the emergency treatment of supraventricular tachycardia. Resuscitation 2009;80:523–8.
75. Alabed S, Sabouni A, Providencia R, et al. Adenosine versus intravenous calcium channel antagonists for supraventricular tachycardia. Cochrane Database Syst Rev 2017;10:CD005154.
76. Delaney B, Loy J, Kelly A-M. The relative efficacy of adenosine versus verapamil for the treatment of stable paroxysmal supraventricular tachycardia in adults: a meta-analysis. Eur J Emerg Med 2011;18:148–52.
77. Ahmad F, Abu Sneineh M, Patel RS, et al. In the line of treatment: a systematic review of paroxysmal supraventricular tachycardia. Cureus 2021;13:e15502.
78. Rankin AC, Brooks R, Ruskin JN, et al. Adenosine and the treatment of supraventricular tachycardia. Am J Med 1992;92:655–64.
79. Riksen NP, Smits P, Rongen GA. The cardiovascular effects of methylxanthines. Handb Exp Pharmacol 2011;200:413–37.

80. Stone PH, Antman EM, Muller JE, et al. Calcium channel blocking agents in the treatment of cardiovascular disorders. Part II: Hemodynamic effects and clinical applications. Ann Intern Med 1980;93:886–904.

81. Moser LR, Smythe MA, Tisdale JE. The use of calcium salts in the prevention and management of verapamil-induced hypotension. Ann Pharmacother 2000;34:622–9.

82. Home, Crediblemeds. Available at: http://www.crediblemeds.org. Accessed December 6, 2021.

83. Redfern WS, Carlsson L, Davis AS, et al. Relationships between preclinical cardiac electrophysiology, clinical QT interval prolongation and torsade de pointes for a broad range of drugs: evidence for a provisional safety margin in drug development. Cardiovasc Res 2003;58:32–45.

84. Yang T, Chun YW, Stroud DM, et al. Screening for acute IKr block is insufficient to detect torsades de pointes liability: role of late sodium current. Circulation 2014;130:224–34.

85. Zeltser D, Justo D, Halkin A, et al. Torsade de pointes due to noncardiac drugs: most patients have easily identifiable risk factors. Medicine 2003;82:282–90.

86. Thomas SHL, Behr ER. Pharmacological treatment of acquired QT prolongation and torsades de pointes. Br J Clin Pharmacol 2016;81:420–7.

87. Al-Khatib SM, Stevenson WG, Ackerman MJ, et al. 2017 AHA/ACC/HRS guideline for management of patients with ventricular arrhythmias and the prevention of sudden cardiac death: a report of the American college of cardiology/American Heart Association Task Force on clinical practice guidelines and the heart rhythm society. Circulation 2018;138:e272–391.

88. Inoue H, Matsuo H, Mashima S, et al. Effects of atrial pacing, isoprenaline and lignocaine on experimental polymorphous ventricular tachycardia. Cardiovasc Res 1984;18:538–47.

89. Wang W-Q, Robertson C, Dhalla AK, et al. Antitorsadogenic effects of ({+/-})-N-(2,6-dimethyl-phenyl)-(4[2-hydroxy-3-(2-methoxyphenoxy)propyl]-1-piperazine (ranolazine) in anesthetized rabbits. J Pharmacol Exp Ther 2008;325:875–81.

90. Assimes TL, Malcolm I. Torsade de pointes with sotalol overdose treated successfully with lidocaine. Can J Cardiol 1998;14:753–6.

91. Takahashi N, Ito M, Inoue T, et al. Torsades de pointes associated with acquired long QT syndrome: observation of 7 cases. J Cardiol 1993;23:99–106.

92. Panchal AR, Bartos JA, Cabañas JG, et al. Part 3: Adult Basic and Advanced Life Support: 2020 American Heart Association Guidelines for Cardiopulmonary Resuscitation and Emergency Cardiovascular Care. Circulation 2020;142:S366–468.

93. Considine J, Gazmuri RJ, Perkins GD, et al. Chest compression components (rate, depth, chest wall recoil and leaning): A scoping review. Resuscitation 2020;146:188–202.

94. Holmberg MJ, Issa MS, Moskowitz A, et al. Vasopressors during adult cardiac arrest: A systematic review and meta-analysis. Resuscitation 2019;139:106–21.

95. Jacobs IG, Finn JC, Jelinek GA, et al. Effect of adrenaline on survival in out-of-hospital cardiac arrest: A randomised double-blind placebo-controlled trial. Resuscitation 2011;82:1138–43.

96. Perkins GD, Ji C, Deakin CD, et al. A randomized trial of epinephrine in out-of-hospital cardiac arrest. N Engl J Med 2018;379:711–21.

97. Dorian P, Cass D, Schwartz B, et al. Amiodarone as compared with lidocaine for shock-resistant ventricular fibrillation. N Engl J Med 2002;346:884–90.

98. Kudenchuk PJ, Cobb LA, Copass MK, et al. Amiodarone for resuscitation after out-of-hospital cardiac arrest due to ventricular fibrillation. N Engl J Med 1999; 341:871–8.

99. Kudenchuk PJ, Brown SP, Daya M, et al. Amiodarone, lidocaine, or placebo in out-of-hospital cardiac arrest. N Engl J Med 2016;374:1711–22.

100. Granfeldt A, Avis SR, Lind PC, et al. Intravenous vs. intraosseous administration of drugs during cardiac arrest: A systematic review. Resuscitation 2020;149: 150–7.

101. Driver BE, Debaty G, Plummer DW, et al. Use of esmolol after failure of standard cardiopulmonary resuscitation to treat patients with refractory ventricular fibrillation. Resuscitation 2014;85:1337–41.

102. Lee YH, Lee KJ, Min YH, et al. Refractory ventricular fibrillation treated with esmolol. Resuscitation 2016;107:150–5.

103. Ortiz M, Martín A, Arribas F, et al. Randomized comparison of intravenous procainamide vs. intravenous amiodarone for the acute treatment of tolerated wide QRS tachycardia: the PROCAMIO study. Eur Heart J 2017;38:1329–35.

104. Gorgels AP, van den Dool A, Hofs A, et al. Comparison of procainamide and lidocaine in terminating sustained monomorphic ventricular tachycardia. Am J Cardiol 1996;78:43–6.

105. Marill KA, deSouza IS, Nishijima DK, et al. Amiodarone or procainamide for the termination of sustained stable ventricular tachycardia: an historical multicenter comparison. Acad Emerg Med 2010;17:297–306.

106. Komura S, Chinushi M, Furushima H, et al. Efficacy of procainamide and lidocaine in terminating sustained monomorphic ventricular tachycardia. Circ J 2010;74:864–9.

Emergency Considerations of Infective Endocarditis

Jobin Philip, MD[1], Michael C. Bond, MD*

KEYWORDS

- Endocarditis • Fever • Murmur • Injection drug use • Bacteremia
- Blood stream infections

KEY POINTS

- The incidence of infective endocarditis (IE) is increasing due to the increased implantation of intracardiac devices, indwelling intravenous lines, and invasive procedures.
- *Staphylococcus aureus* has become the most common pathogen worldwide. Further, *S aureus* is the leading cause of health care associated IE, with many of the cases being methicillin-resistant *S aureus*.
- Despite appropriate antibiotic therapy, approximately 50% of patients will still require surgery.
- The modified Duke criteria now includes alternative imaging findings on computed tomography (CT) or PET/CT (eg, abnormal activity around prosthetic valves, paravalvular lesions) as major criteria for IE.
- Prophylactic antibiotics before procedures are needed only in high-risk individuals (ie, patients with prosthetic valves, previous episodes of IE, or congenital heart disease).

INTRODUCTION

Infective endocarditis (IE) is an uncommon infection that affects the endocardial surface of the heart, most commonly the heart valves (native or prosthetic). Still, it can also occur on mural endocardium septal defects and in-dwelling cardiac devices. Although uncommon, these infections can have devastating health consequences if the diagnosis is delayed or missed. The incidence of IE is increasing due to the increased use of intracardiac devices and indwelling intravenous (IV) lines, along with the number of invasive procedures that patients undergo that increase their risk of transient bacteremia. All patients with a fever and no localizing source should be risk-stratified for the possibility of IE. However, IE is not just limited to individuals with an IV drug use (IVDU) history, but must also be considered in those that have

Department of Emergency Medicine, University of Maryland School of Medicine, 110 South Paca Street, Sixth Floor, Suite 200, Baltimore, MD 21201, USA
[1] Present address: 1001 Monroe Avenue Northwest, Apartment 303, Grand Rapids, MI 49503.
* Corresponding author.
E-mail address: mbond@som.umaryland.edu

Emerg Med Clin N Am 40 (2022) 793–808
https://doi.org/10.1016/j.emc.2022.07.001
0733-8627/22/© 2022 Elsevier Inc. All rights reserved.

had recent infections or dental procedures, have indwelling IV lines or cardiac devices, are on dialysis, or had recent surgical procedures.

EPIDEMIOLOGY

The annual incidence of IE is estimated to be 3–10/100,000 per year in developed countries and has not changed significantly over the last two decades.[1] Historically, viridians group Streptococci was the most common pathogen causing IE, but during the previous 20 years, Staphylococcus aureus has become the most common pathogen worldwide.[2] Further, S aureus is the leading cause of health care associated IE, with many cases being methicillin-resistant S aureus (MRSA). Infrequent etiologies of IE are due to a group of Gram-negative bacilli known as HACEK (non-Influenzae hemophilus, Aggregatibacter, Cardiobacterium, Eikenella, and Kingella). They have a much lower incidence of 1.2/1,000,000 persons per year.[3] A Mayo clinic study showed the mean age of patients with IE has changed over the years, from 65 years in 1970–74, to 46.5 years in 1980–84, to 70 years in 1995–2006.[4] The incidence in women has also increased from 2% in 1970–74 to 50% in 2001–2006.[4] This was further confirmed in a study out of Belgium that showed that the average age of onset of IE has increased from 35 years to 50 years; they also noted that women had twice the incidence of IE than men.[5]

Rheumatic heart disease (RHD) has historically been a major risk factor for IE, but the incidence of RHD is very low in developed countries. RHD remains the leading risk factor in low-income countries.[6,7] In developed countries predisposing risk factors include IVDU, cardiac devices [eg, pacemakers, automatic implantable cardioverter-defibrillators, stents, and transcatheter aortic valve replacement (TAVR)], congenital heart disease, degenerative valve disease, and prosthetic valves.[8] The increased use of cardiac devices has caused an increase in the incidence of prosthetic valve and cardiac device-related endocarditis, from 12% to 13.8% and 1.3% to 4.1%, respectively.[9] Native valve IE (NVE) still accounts for the majority (71%–78%) of cases; 5% to 13% of cases are IVDU related.[9–11] One meta-analysis showed the overall incidence of IE after TAVR was 7/1000 patients per year, and these patients had a pooled mortality rate of 39%.[12]

Health care associated infections have been shown to account for half of the cases of NVE in one US study[9]; however, another French study showed the incidence was only 26.7%.[13] Regardless, health care associated infections result in significant disability, prolonged hospitalizations, increased costs, and an associated mortality rate as high as 50% at one year.[9] Due to dedicated efforts to decrease catheter-related bloodstream infections, there has been a significant decrease in nosocomial IE cases.

PATHOPHYSIOLOGY

Endocarditis is defined as an infection of the endocardial surface of the heart, which comprises four chambers and four valves. Endocarditis can involve the endocardial surface, valvular structures, or a pre-existing intracardiac device. Endocarditis can be the result of endocardial injury (from lines and intracardiac devices), turbulent flow (eg, atrial septal defects, ventricle septal defects) that all result in the development of a fibrin clot that allows for bacterial adherence and overgrowth. Valve leaflet distortion and destruction lead to regurgitant flow, impaired cardiac function, and heart failure, which is the leading cause of death in patients with IE.[14] The heart valve most commonly affected is the mitral valve, followed by the aortic valve, tricuspid valve, and rarely the pulmonic valve.

COMPLICATIONS/CONCERNS

IE is associated with several severe sequelae that can complicate treatment decisions, as the provider tries to optimize treatment while preventing additional complications. These complications can occur due to the destruction of the heart valves, the development of abscesses in the heart, or the result of embolization of vegetation to distal sites. Systemic septic emboli are more common with left-side IE with the brain and spleen being the most frequent sites. Factors associated with increased risk of septic emboli are noted in Factors Associated with Increased Risk of Septic Emboli[15,16]

- Size (>10 mm) and mobility of vegetations (most potent independent predictors)
- Mitral valve location
- *S aureus, S bovis, Candida* spp
- History of previous embolism
- Multivalvular IE

Potential complications of IE are shown in **Table 1**.[17–19]

Cardiac

The most frequent complication of IE is heart failure, which occurs in up to 70% of patients with IE.[14] Congestive Heart Failure (CHF) is often due to incompetence of the aortic valve resulting in serve aortic regurgitation, which is the most common indication for surgery.[20–22] Mitral regurgitation and intracardiac fistulas can also lead to heart failure. Mitral valve infection can lead to rupture of chordae tendineae or papillary muscles. Patients with elevated left atrial pressure, moderate-to-severe pulmonary hypertension, or elevated left ventricular end-diastolic pressure are also candidates for surgery even if they do not clinically have heart failure.[23–25]

Vegetations can also embolize into a coronary artery causing myocardial ischemia. These patients need to be closely managed in collaboration with cardiology as anticoagulation can increase their risk of rupture of mycotic aneurysms. Myocarditis and pericarditis are also possible. Myocarditis can be secondary to abscess formation or an immune reaction.

Atrioventricular blocks are estimated to occur in between 1% and 15% of cases. Often, these blocks are associated with perivalvular abscesses or fistulas around the aortic or mitral valves.[26]

Table 1	
Complications of infective endocarditis[17–19]	
- Cardiac	- Musculoskeletal
○ Congestive heart failure	○ Arthritis
○ Atrioventricular blocks	○ Myositis
○ Valvular insufficiency	○ Abscesses
○ Myocardial infarction	○ Septic joint
○ Cardiac arrhythmias	- Renal
○ Aortic root or myocardial abscesses	○ Acute kidney failure
○ Pericarditis	○ Glomerulonephritis
- Neurologic	○ Renal infarction
○ Stroke: ischemic or hemorrhagic	- Mesenteric
○ Cerebral abscess	○ Splenic abscess
○ Spinal epidural abscess	○ Mesenteric ischemia
○ Mycotic aneurysm	- Pulmonary
	○ Septic emboli

Patients who have evidence of persistent infections (positive blood cultures after 7–10 days) need to be evaluated for perivalvular extension and abscess formation. The perivalvular extension is more common in aortic valve IE, in patients with prosthetic valves, and when the causative agent is coagulase-negative *Staphylococcus*.[27–29] Even with surgical repair, these patients have a hospital mortality rate estimated at 40%.[30–32] These patients may also develop ventricular septal defects, atrioventricular blocks, and acute coronary syndrome.[32–34]

Neurologic

It is estimated that symptomatic neurological complications (eg, stroke, brain abscess, meningitis, encephalopathy) occur in 15%–30% of patients with IE.[35,36] Several studies have shown that 35%–60% of IE patients have clinically silent cerebral embolisms.[37,38] A stroke may be the presenting symptom in some patients and standard treatment (ie, anticoagulation) can increase the patient's risk for intracranial bleeds and rupture of mycotic aneurysms. As expected, these complications are associated with increased mortality. In patients with IE, early initiation of appropriate antibiotics is the most important factor in preventing additional sequelae.[39] Neither stroke nor an intracranial hemorrhage is an absolute contraindication to surgery if the patient is expected to have a good recovery.[40] Emergency medicine physicians should consider IE and septic emboli as a cause of a patient's acute neurological presentation if they are noted to have new murmurs, a history of IE, fever, or risk factors for IE. This concern should be relayed to the admitting and consulting services to perform an appropriate risk/benefits analysis before anticoagulants or thrombolytic agents are given.

Mycotic aneurysms can occur anywhere in the body and have variable clinical presentations. Seeding of the vessel's walls causes the vessel to become thin-walled and friable with an increased risk of rupture and subsequent hemorrhage. Intracranial ruptures are the most frequent and estimated to occur in 2%–4% of IE patients.[41,42] The clinical presentation is variable, and patients can present with altered mental status, headache, hemorrhagic stroke, or seizures. Computed tomography (CT) of the head without contrast can visualize the intracranial bleeding while a CT angiogram has good sensitivity and specificity in detecting aneurysms and helping to determine if neurosurgical or endovascular therapy would be beneficial.

Musculoskeletal

Patients with IE can also develop musculoskeletal complaints to include myalgias (12%–15%) and back pain (13% of IE cases).[43,44] Pain in the lumbar spine is the most common location. Back pain can be benign or a marker of a more serious infection, such as a spinal epidural abscess (SEA) or osteomyelitis. It is estimated that vertebral osteomyelitis occurs in 5%–19% of patients with IE.[43] If SEA is suspected an MRI with a contrast of the entire spine is needed as skip lesions are common, and the location of the pain is not predictive of the location of an abscess.

Mesenteric

Splenic infarcts are very common but often asymptomatic and are usually incidental findings on abdominal CTs. For patients with signs of persistent infections, an abdominal CT is useful to ascertain whether there is a splenic abscess or rupture. Large splenic abscesses may need to be treated surgically or with percutaneous drainage. However, most cases are treated with appropriate antibiotics.

Renal

Acute renal failure (ARF) occurs in 6%–30% of patients with IE and is associated with increased mortality and morbidity. The causes of ARF in IE patients are shown in Causes of Acute Renal Failure in IE.[41]

- Immune complex deposition
- Glomerulonephritis
- Renal infarction secondary to septic emboli
- Renal impairment due to hemodynamic instability/hypotension secondary to sepsis
- Antibiotic toxicity
- Nephrotoxicity secondary to contrast agents

To minimize the risk of ARF, antibiotics should be renally dosed and therapeutic levels monitored, exposure to radiologic contrast should be minimized, mean arterial blood pressure maintained, and adequate IV fluids should be provided to prevent pre-renal failure.

Pulmonary

Right-sided vegetations tend to produce septic pulmonary emboli.[45]

CLINICAL FEATURES

IE is a challenging diagnosis that is often missed on the first clinical encounter because its clinical presentation is very diverse and nonspecific. This often delays definitive management and contributes to the mortality of IE. However, IE should be considered in anyone with sepsis of unknown origin or fever in the presence of risk factors Risk Factors for IE.[47,48]

- Congenital heart disease
- Hemodialysis
- History of endocarditis
- Immunosuppression
- Implanted heart device
- Intravenous drug use
- Long-term catheter use
- Poor dental health
- Prosthetic valve replacement
- Pulmonary hypertension
- Recent dental or surgical procedure
- Rheumatic heart disease

The disease course is influenced by host factors, location of the vegetation, and microbial virulence resulting in a wide range of presentations: from indolent infection with nonspecific symptoms in a well-appearing patient to acute, severe infection presenting as septic shock and multiorgan failure.

Patients with acute IE develop the rapidly progressive disease in the form of rigors, sepsis, and systemic manifestations, whereas those with subacute (develops over weeks to months) IE present with more vague and chronic symptoms.[46] IE can also present with one of its complications, particularly stroke or systemic embolisms. No matter the presentation, patients with persistent unexplained bacteremia should be investigated for IE.

The initial clinical assessment of a patient with suspected IE involves an evaluation of risk factors (List 3) and a search for a supportive history and examination findings.[47,48] Major cardiac risk factors are a prior history of IE, a prosthetic valve or cardiac device, and valvular or congenital heart disease. Noncardiac risk factors are IVDU, dialysis, indwelling IV lines, immunosuppression, or a recent dental or surgical procedure.

Fever is the most commonly reported symptom and is seen in 90% of patients.[6] Fever also represents one of the minor Duke criteria.[49] However, fever may have varying patterns or even be absent, especially in the elderly, the immunosuppressed, and those with recent antibiotic or antipyretic use. Other constitutional symptoms are nonspecific and may include myalgias, weight loss, anorexia, night sweats, headache, dyspnea, cough, and chest pain. These vague symptoms are more common in patients who present subacutely.

Cardiac murmurs are the most common examination finding and are observed in 85% of patients.[6] Other supportive examination findings include splenomegaly, petechiae, and splinter hemorrhages. Classic medical teaching emphasizes the presence of Osler's nodes, Roth's spots, and Janeway lesions. While highly specific for IE, these are surprisingly rare, especially in acute cases which may develop other complications too quickly to manifest immunologic vascular findings. Overall, the sensitivity and specificity of any one sign are low. Therefore, a normal physical examination should not be used to exclude the diagnosis of IE.

IE can also present with a complication (see **Table 1**). In 30% of cases, patients' initial presenting symptom is related to heart failure, paravalvular abscess formation, embolic stroke, or other metastatic infection, including vertebral osteomyelitis or peripheral abscesses. Complications of IE can ultimately involve any organ system or can be related to a systemic/embolic infection.

EVALUATION/DIAGNOSIS

The diagnosis of IE requires a high index of suspicion and should be considered in all patients with fever and new cardiac murmur, sepsis of unclear etiology, or underlying IE risk factors. The diagnosis of IE is ultimately made by a combination of clinical findings (as described earlier), microbiological data from blood cultures, and echocardiogram.

Microbiology/Blood Cultures

Positive blood cultures are important for the diagnosis of IE and are a major Duke criterion. Three sets of blood cultures (20 mL each) can detect 96%–98% of bacteremia cases and should be obtained before the initiation of IV antibiotics. Ideally, cultures should be drawn from three separate venipuncture sites at least 30 to 60 minutes apart to limit and help distinguish skin contaminants from genuine bacteremia.[50] Some investigators have argued that two sets are adequate in most situations. Three sets are mandatory in suspected prosthetic valve IE (PVE), because one of the most common pathogens, coagulase-negative *Staphylococcus*, is also the most common blood culture contaminant.[45]

Gram-positive cocci account for the majority of cases of IE. *Staphylococcus* species are most frequently isolated, with *S aureus* the most common organism, causing 20%–68% of cases in both native and prosthetic valve infections, and these patients should be examined with echocardiography.[6,51,52] MRSA is becoming an increasing problem, especially among high-risk groups, such as IVDUs, chronic hemodialysis patients, and patients with contact with health care providers. Compared with other pathogens, *S aureus* IE carries an increased rate of complications, including embolic disease, abscess formation, and higher in-hospital and 30-day mortality risk.[45]

Coagulase-negative *Staphylococci* (*S epidermidis, S lugdunensis,* and *S capitis,* frequently found on skin) have lower virulence potential than *S aureus* but greater ability to adhere to prosthetic material due to its biofilm production. These species cause 17% of early PVE and frequently infect indwelling catheters and devices.[6] The other gram-positive cocci that are common causes of IE are the viridans group *Streptococci* (VGS) sp (*S mutans, S salivarius, S anginosus, S mitis,* and *S sanguinis*) and *Enterococcus* species. VGS infection remains common in community-acquired NVE and accounts for a higher proportion of disease in developing countries. This group comes from the oral, gastrointestinal, and genitourinary tract and is typically less virulent than *S aureus*. There is a significant incidence of VGS infections in the IVDU population due to the practice of using saliva to clean needles and dissolve heroin, thus introducing oral bacteria into the bloodstream. Group D *Streptococci* (*S bovis* and *S equinus* complex) cause IE associated with underlying colon cancer and advanced liver disease. *Enterococcal* IE tends to be indolent and is associated with underlying valve disease, older age, and chronic illness. *Enterococcus* isolates are increasingly resistant to vancomycin, aminoglycosides, and ampicillin.[6]

The remaining common IE pathogens include a mixture of fastidious, zoonotic, and intracellular bacteria and fungi that often result in persistently negative blood cultures (culture-negative endocarditis). The HACEK group is slow-growing bacteria of the oropharynx, associated with periodontal disease, and have long been recognized as potential causes of both NVE and PVE. Zoonotic bacteria that cause IE are mostly intracellular pathogens and include *Coxiella burnetii* from livestock, *Bartonella henselae* from cats, and *Chlamydia psittaci* from parrots and pigeons. *Tropheryma whippelii, Legionella* sp, *Mycoplasma* sp, and *Pseudomonas aeruginosa* are other rare causes of IE. Fungal causes of IE include *Candida* and *Aspergillus* and are a rare but significant cause of IE in immunocompromised patients and those with prosthetic valves.[53]

About 10% of patients with IE show no growth from blood cultures, which can prevent diagnosis. Several causes can account for this: antibiotics given before blood cultures, infection with fastidious bacteria or fungi, or alternative diagnoses, such as nonbacterial thrombotic endocarditis, which occurs in advanced cancer.[54] In some emergency department (ED) cases, antibiotics will have been administered before the diagnosis of IE is considered. In such cases, blood cultures should still be drawn because they retain a reasonable sensitivity for bacteremia even after antibiotics have been administered.

A causative organism can be identified in about two-thirds of patients by further microbiological testing.[55] If cultures are negative at 5 days, serological testing for *Coxiella* and *Bartonella* should be done. If negative, testing for *Brucella, Mycoplasma, Legionella,* and *Chlamydia* should be undertaken. Extended blood culture after 7 days provides no further useful yield, even for the HACEK bacteria.[6]

Echocardiography

An echocardiogram is key to the diagnosis of IE and is one of the modified major Duke criteria. Abnormal findings include valvular vegetations, perivalvular abscesses, or leaflet perforations. Transthoracic echocardiogram (TTE) has a sensitivity of 70% for diagnosing NVE and 50% for PVE.[41] Despite its low sensitivity, TTE has a high negative predictive value; therefore, it should be the initial imaging study of choice in patients with suspected IE. The sensitivity of TTE is higher in IVDU-related cases because vegetations are larger and right-sided, and these younger patients often have a smaller body habitus.[56]

Transesophageal echocardiogram (TEE) is more sensitive (sensitivity of more than 90%) than TTE. TEE is preferred over TTE in patients with a known prosthetic valve, intracardiac implant, or intracardiac abscess. TEE is also more sensitive in identifying clinically important complications, such as paravalvular abscess, valve prolapse, valve leaflet perforation, pseudoaneurysm, torn chordae tendineae, and vegetations on pacemaker wires.[57]

Patients with a high clinical suspicion for IE and a negative or equivocal TTE should still undergo TEE. A three-dimensional TEE allows visualization of the affected valve in multiple planes to diagnose leaflet perforation and guide surgical planning. A normal TEE strongly predicts the absence of disease, but a repeat study should be done 7–10 days later if clinical suspicion is high. If the repeat study is negative, further echocardiography rarely brings additional value. The specificity of echocardiography is not 100% and false-positive cases can occur with cardiac tumors, thrombi, and fibrous strands on the aortic valve.

Echocardiography also provides information on the hemodynamic severity of the valve lesion and the underlying left- and right ventricular function, which may be helpful in determining if surgery is indicated. Cardiac surgery may be indicated for a vegetation diameter greater than 10 mm as well as for other echocardiographic findings, such as severe valvular insufficiency, intracardiac abscess, pseudoaneurysm, valvular perforation or dehiscence, and decompensated CHF.[27]

OTHER DIAGNOSTIC TESTING
Electrocardiogram

An electrocardiogram (ECG) may show new conduction disorders, such as first-degree atrioventricular block, bundle branch block, or complete heart block, indicating the extension of infection into the His–Purkinje system. The ECG may also demonstrate cardiac ischemia in the rare case of coronary artery emboli.[14]

Laboratory Studies

Early laboratory studies are generally nonspecific and should not be used to rule out IE. An elevated white blood cell level is nonspecific and is typically seen in 50% of cases. Elevated inflammatory markers (C-reactive protein and erythrocyte sedimentation rate) have been reported in up to 66% of cases. Serum lactate and other tests of impaired organ perfusion should be routinely obtained along with blood cultures. Given the typical and atypical presentations of IE, a broad diagnostic workup is often ordered initially and there are several laboratory abnormalities that, although nonspecific, may suggest the correct diagnosis.

Newer molecular methods, such as polymerase chain reaction and DNA microarray assays, are being investigated. These may detect bacteremia and identify the pathogen in a matter of hours, rather than relying on blood cultures, which can take days. More extensive clinical trials are required, but these methods hold great promise for rapidly detecting bacteremia and determining antibiotic resistance patterns in the future.[58–60]

Imaging

The chest radiograph is frequently abnormal in right-sided IE as septic pulmonary emboli may appear as peripheral, poorly marginated nodules, predominantly occurring in the lower lobes. This may be mistaken for multifocal pneumonia. In severe left-sided infection, the chest radiograph reveals signs of CHF.[61] Newer imaging modalities are being used for further evaluation of IE and its complications. Cardiac CT or coronary CT angiography may improve the evaluation of paravalvular complications, such as abscesses or aneurysms before surgery. Although cardiac CT angiography has excellent spatial resolution and less imaging artifact from the prosthetic valve than TEE, it is less sensitive than TEE for detecting small vegetations. Cardiac MRI can distinguish vegetations from tumors. Brain MRI has a role in identifying cerebral emboli and mycotic aneurysms. Radionuclide studies, including PET-CT, have also been used to detect peripheral embolization and both cardiac and extracardiac sites of infection by finding infectious foci that are metabolically active and readily take up radionuclide glucose tracer.[6,27]

Modified Duke criteria

The Duke criteria were originally developed for scientific research classification and not as a clinical instrument.[49] It has reduced sensitivity in patients with suspected PVE, right-sided IE, and cardiac device infection. The main utility in the emergency setting is to provide a checklist of key historical and examination features to consider and serve as a reminder of the importance of blood cultures. The modified Duke criteria use pathologic, clinical, and microbiologic data elements to diagnose IE.[62] It was recently updated by the European Society of Cardiology (ESC) to recommend that a paravalvular lesion seen on cardiac CT or the presence of abnormal activity around the site of implantation of a prosthetic value > 3 months after surgery on an ^{18}F-FDG PET/CT be considered a major criterion and that recent embolic events or infectious aneurysms by imaging only (silent events) should be considered a minor criterion.[41] The ESC modified Duke criteria are shown in **Table 1**. Diagnosis of IE is definite in the presence of two major criteria, or one major and three minor criteria, or five minor criteria; or diagnosis of IE is possible in the presence of one major and one minor criterion, or three minor criteria (**Box 1**).

TREATMENT

The treatment of IE in the ED begins with an evaluation of clinical stability. When patients present with hypotension and shock, it is important to resuscitate and manage both septic shock and cardiogenic shock appropriately. When approaching a critical patient, initial management should focus on obtaining early blood cultures and administering antibiotics while providing the appropriate and necessary hemodynamic support. A bedside echocardiogram or urgent/emergent TTE should be performed to assess for complications of IE that may require cardiothoracic surgery.

In a clinically stable patient with possible NVE, it is reasonable for the clinician to defer antibiotics while awaiting blood culture results. However, it is important to maintain a high index of suspicion for IE in all febrile patients with risk factors to avoid delays in the diagnosis and reduce the risk of morbidity and mortality. The treatment of IE requires a multidisciplinary approach and includes IV antibiotics and potentially further source control with early surgery. Despite appropriate treatment with early IV antibiotics, 50% of patients will still require surgery to replace the infected valve or drain intracardiac abscesses.[63]

Antibiotics

Antibiotic selection for IE is a complex topic. The antibiotics should be bactericidal and tailored to the treatment of *Staphylococci*, *Streptococci*, and *Enterococci* in both NVE and PVE, but should also cover MRSA in PVE. Most regimens also provide coverage for the beta-lactamase-producing HACEK organisms.

Recommendations vary as to when to cover MRSA in NVE. Some US experts recommend empirically covering MRSA in all cases, regardless of risk factors.[64] In general, vancomycin can be given in the ED as an initial empiric therapy. In patients who cannot tolerate vancomycin, daptomycin is a good alternative, with recent

---

Box 1
ECS 2015-modified criteria for the diagnosis of infective endocarditis[41]

Major Criteria
I. I. Blood cultures positive for IE
   A. Typical microorganisms consistent with IE from two separate blood cultures:
      1. Viridans streptococci, *Streptococcus gallolyticus* (*S bovis*), HACEK group, *S aureus*; or
      2. Community-acquired enterococci, in the absence of a primary focus; or
   B. Microorganisms consistent with IE from persistently positive blood cultures:
      1. ≥2 positive blood cultures of blood samples drawn >12 h apart; or
      2. All of 3 or a majority of 24 separate cultures of blood (with first and last samples drawn ≥1 h apart); or
   C. Single positive blood culture for *Coxiella burnetii* or phase IgG antibody titer >1:800
1. Imaging positive for IE
   a. Echocardiogram positive for IE:
      i. Vegetations
      ii. Abscess, pseudoaneurysm, intracardiac fistula;
      iii. Valvular perforation or aneurysm;
      iv. New partial dehiscence of prosthetic valve.
   b. Abnormal activity around the site of prosthetic valve implantation detected by ^{18}F-FDG PET/CT (only if the prosthesis was implanted for >3 months) or radiolabeled leukocytes SPECT/CT.
   c. Definite paravalvular lesions by cardiac CT

Minor Criteria
1. Predisposition, such as predisposing heart condition, or injection drug use
2. Fever defined as temperature >38°C
3. Vascular phenomena (including those detected by imaging only): major arterial emboli, septic pulmonary infarcts, infectious (mycotic) aneurysm, intracranial hemorrhage, conjunctival hemorrhages, and Janeway's lesions
4. Immunological phenomena: glomerulonephritis, Osler's nodes, Roth's spots, and rheumatoid factor
5. Microbiological evidence: positive blood culture but does not meet a major criterion as noted earlier or serological evidence of active infection with organism consistent with IE

Abbreviations: CT, computed tomography; FDG, fluorodeoxyglucose; HACEK *Haemophilus parainfluenzae, H aphrophilus, H paraphrophilus, H influenzae, Actinobacillus actinomycetemcomitans, Cardiobacterium hominis, Eikenella corrodens, Kingella kingae,* and *K denitrificans;* IE, infective endocarditis; Ig, immunoglobulin; SPECT, single-photon emission computerized tomography.

Adapted from Li et al.[62]

---

studies concluding that it is noninferior against *S aureus*, including MRSA, and *Streptococcus* sp.[65]

Whether *Pseudomonas* and highly resistant *Enterobacteriaceae* strains should be covered immediately in certain patients (eg, IVDU, recent invasive procedure) is controversial. Aminoglycosides are recommended in many regimens because they have a synergistic effect with beta-lactams and vancomycin, providing enhanced bactericidal activity, particularly against *Enterococcus*. However, nephrotoxicity concerns and dosing difficulties arise beyond the first dose; in addition to a lack of mortality benefit. Likewise, rifampin appears in empiric regimens for suspected PVE because it may be beneficial against MRSA and coagulase-negative *Staphylococci* in this setting. Nonetheless, its use is also controversial because of concerns for the rapid development of resistance, hepatotoxicity, and drug interaction problems.[45]

Antibiotics can be modified and narrowed according to culture results, resistance patterns, the severity of infection, and the presence or absence of prosthetic material. Hospital-specific empiric treatment recommendations are often preferred over published guidelines because they account for local susceptibility patterns and are developed by local infectious disease specialists.

Current guidelines recommend that patients with IE undergo treatment with IV antibiotics for 6 weeks. A recent randomized, noninferiority, multicenter trial found that clinically stable patients with left-sided IE treated with oral antibiotics compared to IV antibiotics had similar outcomes in mortality.[66] The results of this trial have not changed current management guidelines but may impact future long-term management.

Surgical Intervention

Despite appropriate antibiotic therapy, approximately 50% of patients with IE (native or prosthetic valve) will still require surgery. **Table 2** lists the indications for surgery. In general, surgery is considered for decompensated heart failure, conduction blocks, or persistent infection that cannot be cleared with antibiotics alone.

Prognosis

Most patients with IE do well with a 5-year survival rate estimated at 60%–70%.[67–69] Patients with CHF, comorbidities, recurrences, or older age are at increased risk of mortality. To improve long-term outcomes and decrease recurrences, patients should be followed closely by cardiology. Patients should also be educated on good dental hygiene, preventive dentistry, and skin hygiene to minimize transient bacteremia that could cause a reoccurrence.

Prevention

In the past, it was routinely recommended that individuals with structural or congenital heart disease receive prophylactic antibiotics before dental and other procedures to prevent IE. However, in 2002, those recommendations changed that only those individuals with the highest risk of IE (ie, patients with prosthetic valves, previous episode

Table 2 Indications for surgery[27]	
Indications for surgery (based on observational studies rather than formal guidelines)	• Valvular dysfunction resulting in acute decompensated heart failure • Heart failure secondary to valve dehiscence, intracardiac fistula, or severe prosthetic valve dysfunction • Infection causing heart block, annular or aortic abscess, or a destructive penetrating lesion • Persistent bacteremia or fever >5–7 d after the initiation of IV antibiotics
Surgery should be considered in the following cases	• Infective endocarditis caused by a fungal infection or a resistant organism • Recurrent emboli or persistent/enlarging vegetations despite IV antibiotics • Severe valvular regurgitation and vegetations >10 mm in size • Vegetations >10 mm when associated with the anterior leaflet of the mitral valve • Relapsing prosthetic valve endocarditis

of IE, or congenital heart disease) or at the highest risk of adverse outcomes from IE should receive antibiotics when they are having a dental procedure requiring the manipulation of the gingival or periapical region of the teeth or perforation of the oral mucosa. It is also recommended that piercings and tattoos be discouraged in these high-risk individuals. Prophylactic treatment is not indicated for respiratory, gastrointestinal, urogenital, or skin/soft tissue procedures. The reason for the changes in prophylactic treatment is that the incidence of IE after these procedures is very low and antibiotic administration increased the risk of the emergence of resistant organisms.[70] Also, the efficacy of antibiotic prophylaxis was only seen in animal models.[71] When indicated, those with high risk should take a single 2 g dose of amoxicillin or ampicillin 30 to 60 minutes before their procedure, or 600 mg of clindamycin if they are penicillin-allergic.

SUMMARY

IE is a rare bacterial infection that involves the heart valves and leads to increased mortality and morbidity. The diagnosis of IE is challenging and requires a high level of suspicion to initiate the appropriate investigation and treatment. Therefore, it is imperative for the emergency physician to be aware of the various presentations, complications, and risk factors that patients with IE may present with. A multidisciplinary approach is needed in patients presenting with complications from septic emboli and CHF. Early involvement of cardiothoracic surgeons is recommended for patients with CHF, conduction delays, intracardiac abscesses, or large vegetations at risk for embolic complications.

CLINICS CARE POINTS

- Cultures positive for coagulase-negative *Staphylococci* are often felt to be a contaminent as they do have a lower virulence, however, they have a greater ability to adhere to prosthetic material due to their biofilm production and are a significant cause of infection in patients with indwelling catheters and devices.
- Blood cultures can remain negative in 10% of patients with infective endocarditis. This can be due to antibiotics being given prior to the cultures being obtained or infection with fastidious bacteria or fungi.
- Transesophageal echocardiogram (TEE) is much more senstitive that transthoracic echocardiograms (TTE), however, most centers screen with TTEs as they are less invasive and easier to obtain. TEEs, however, maybe needed to help with surgical planning as they are much better at identifying paravalvular abscess, valve prolapse, valve leaflet perforation, pseudoaneurysm, torn chordae tendineae, and vegetations on pacemaker wires.
- The Modified Duke's criteria should be used for diagnosis as it accounts for more advanced imaging techniques that are now available.

DISCLOSURE

The authors have nothing to disclose.

REFERENCES

1. Leone S, Ravasio V, Durante-Mangoni E, et al. Epidemiology, characteristics, and outcome of infective endocarditis in Italy: the Italian Study on Endocarditis. Infection 2012;40(5):527–35.

2. Talha KM, DeSimone DC, Sohail MR, et al. Pathogen influence on epidemiology, diagnostic evaluation and management of infective endocarditis. Heart 2020; 106(24):1878–82.

3. Berge A, Morenius C, Petropoulos A, et al. Epidemiology, bacteriology, and clinical characteristics of HACEK bacteremia and endocarditis: a population-based retrospective study. Eur J Clin Microbiol Infect Dis 2021;40(3):525–34.

4. Correa de Sa DD, Tleyjeh IM, Anavekar NS, et al. Epidemiological trends of infective endocarditis: a population-based study in Olmsted County, Minnesota. Mayo Clin Proc 2010;85(5):422–6.

5. Hill EE, Herijgers P, Claus P, et al. Infective endocarditis: changing epidemiology and predictors of 6-month mortality: a prospective cohort study. Eur Heart J 2007; 28(2):196–203.

6. Cahill TJ, Prendergast BD. Infective endocarditis. Lancet 2016;387(10021): 882–93.

7. Marijon E, Ou P, Celermajer DS, et al. Prevalence of rheumatic heart disease detected by echocardiographic screening. N Engl J Med 2007;357(5):470–6.

8. Tleyjeh IM, Abdel-Latif A, Rahbi H, et al. A systematic review of population-based studies of infective endocarditis. Chest 2007;132(3):1025–35.

9. Toyoda N, Chikwe J, Itagaki S, et al. Trends in infective endocarditis in california and New York state, 1998-2013. JAMA 2017;317(16):1652–60.

10. Habib G, Hoen B, Tornos P, et al. Guidelines on the prevention, diagnosis, and treatment of infective endocarditis (new version 2009): the Task Force on the Prevention, Diagnosis, and Treatment of Infective Endocarditis of the European Society of Cardiology (ESC). Endorsed by the European Society of Clinical Microbiology and Infectious Diseases (ESCMID) and the International Society of Chemotherapy (ISC) for Infection and Cancer. Eur Heart J 2009;30(19): 2369–413.

11. Hoen B, Duval X. Infective endocarditis. N Engl J Med 2013;369(8):785.

12. Prasitlumkum N, Vutthikraivit W, Thangjui S, et al. Epidemiology of infective endocarditis in transcatheter aortic valve replacement: systemic review and meta-analysis. J Cardiovasc Med (Hagerstown) 2020;21(10):790–801.

13. Selton-Suty C, Celard M, Le Moing V, et al. Preeminence of staphylococcus aureus in infective endocarditis: a 1-year population-based survey. Clin Infect Dis 2012;54(9):1230–9.

14. Sexton DJ, Spelman D. Current best practices and guidelines. Assessment and management of complications in infective endocarditis. Infect Dis Clin North Am 2002;16(2):507–21, xii.

15. Thuny F, Di Salvo G, Belliard O, et al. Risk of embolism and death in infective endocarditis: prognostic value of echocardiography: a prospective multicenter study. Circulation 2005;112(1):69–75.

16. Vilacosta I, Graupner C, San Roman JA, et al. Risk of embolization after institution of antibiotic therapy for infective endocarditis. J Am Coll Cardiol 2002;39(9): 1489–95.

17. Conlon PJ, Jefferies F, Krigman HR, et al. Predictors of prognosis and risk of acute renal failure in bacterial endocarditis. Clin Nephrol 1998;49(2):96–101.

18. Fowler RA, Gupta S. Subacute and acute infective endocarditis. Lancet 2005; 366(9501):1964.

19. Weinstein L. Life-threatening complications of infective endocarditis and their management. Arch Intern Med 1986;146(5):953–7.

20. Hasbun R, Vikram HR, Barakat LA, et al. Complicated left-sided native valve endocarditis in adults: risk classification for mortality. JAMA 2003;289(15):1933–40.

21. Nadji G, Rusinaru D, Remadi JP, et al. Heart failure in left-sided native valve infective endocarditis: characteristics, prognosis, and results of surgical treatment. Eur J Heart Fail 2009;11(7):668–75.

22. Olmos C, Vilacosta I, Fernandez C, et al. Comparison of clinical features of left-sided infective endocarditis involving previously normal versus previously abnormal valves. Am J Cardiol 2014;114(2):278–83.

23. Hubert S, Thuny F, Resseguier N, et al. Prediction of symptomatic embolism in infective endocarditis: construction and validation of a risk calculator in a multicenter cohort. J Am Coll Cardiol 2013;62(15):1384–92.

24. Lalani T, Chu VH, Park LP, et al. In-hospital and 1-year mortality in patients undergoing early surgery for prosthetic valve endocarditis. JAMA Intern Med 2013; 173(16):1495–504.

25. Lopez J, Sevilla T, Vilacosta I, et al. Clinical significance of congestive heart failure in prosthetic valve endocarditis. A multicenter study with 257 patients. Rev Esp Cardiol (Engl Ed) 2013;66(5):384–90.

26. DiNubile MJ, Calderwood SB, Steinhaus DM, et al. Cardiac conduction abnormalities complicating native valve active infective endocarditis. Am J Cardiol 1986;58(13):1213–7.

27. Baddour LM, Wilson WR, Bayer AS, et al. Infective endocarditis in adults: diagnosis, antimicrobial therapy, and management of complications: a scientific statement for healthcare professionals from the american heart association. Circulation 2015;132(15):1435–86.

28. Chan KL. Early clinical course and long-term outcome of patients with infective endocarditis complicated by perivalvular abscess. CMAJ 2002;167(1):19–24.

29. Horstkotte D, Follath F, Gutschik E, et al. Guidelines on prevention, diagnosis and treatment of infective endocarditis executive summary; the task force on infective endocarditis of the European society of cardiology. Eur Heart J 2004;25(3): 267–76.

30. Anguera I, Miro JM, Vilacosta I, et al. Aorto-cavitary fistulous tract formation in infective endocarditis: clinical and echocardiographic features of 76 cases and risk factors for mortality. Eur Heart J 2005;26(3):288–97.

31. Bashore TM, Cabell C, Fowler V Jr. Update on infective endocarditis. Curr Probl Cardiol 2006;31(4):274–352.

32. Manzano MC, Vilacosta I, San Roman JA, et al. [Acute coronary syndrome in infective endocarditis]. Rev Esp Cardiol 2007;60(1):24–31.

33. Anguera I, Miro JM, Evangelista A, et al. Periannular complications in infective endocarditis involving native aortic valves. Am J Cardiol 2006;98(9):1254–60.

34. Anguera I, Miro JM, San Roman JA, et al. Periannular complications in infective endocarditis involving prosthetic aortic valves. Am J Cardiol 2006;98(9):1261–8.

35. Garcia-Cabrera E, Fernandez-Hidalgo N, Almirante B, et al. Neurological complications of infective endocarditis: risk factors, outcome, and impact of cardiac surgery: a multicenter observational study. Circulation 2013;127(23):2272–84.

36. Murdoch DR, Corey GR, Hoen B, et al. Clinical presentation, etiology, and outcome of infective endocarditis in the 21st century: the International Collaboration on Endocarditis-Prospective Cohort Study. Arch Intern Med 2009;169(5): 463–73.

37. Hess A, Klein I, Iung B, et al. Brain MRI findings in neurologically asymptomatic patients with infective endocarditis. AJNR Am J Neuroradiol 2013;34(8):1579–84.

38. Snygg-Martin U, Gustafsson L, Rosengren L, et al. Cerebrovascular complications in patients with left-sided infective endocarditis are common: a prospective

study using magnetic resonance imaging and neurochemical brain damage markers. Clin Infect Dis 2008;47(1):23–30.

39. Dickerman SA, Abrutyn E, Barsic B, et al. The relationship between the initiation of antimicrobial therapy and the incidence of stroke in infective endocarditis: an analysis from the ICE Prospective Cohort Study (ICE-PCS). Am Heart J 2007; 154(6):1086–94.

40. Ruttmann E, Willeit J, Ulmer H, et al. Neurological outcome of septic cardioembolic stroke after infective endocarditis. Stroke 2006;37(8):2094–9.

41. Habib G, Lancellotti P, Antunes MJ, et al. 2015 ESC Guidelines for the management of infective endocarditis: The Task Force for the Management of Infective Endocarditis of the European Society of Cardiology (ESC). Endorsed by: European Association for Cardio-Thoracic Surgery (EACTS), the European Association of Nuclear Medicine (EANM). Eur Heart J 2015;36(44):3075–128.

42. Hui FK, Bain M, Obuchowski NA, et al. Mycotic aneurysm detection rates with cerebral angiography in patients with infective endocarditis. J Neurointerv Surg 2015;7(6):449–52.

43. Gonzalez-Juanatey C, Gonzalez-Gay MA, Llorca J, et al. Rheumatic manifestations of infective endocarditis in non-addicts. A 12-year study. Medicine (Baltimore) 2001;80(1):9–19.

44. Pigrau C, Almirante B, Flores X, et al. Spontaneous pyogenic vertebral osteomyelitis and endocarditis: incidence, risk factors, and outcome. Am J Med 2005; 118(11):1287.

45. Yang E, Frazee BW. Infective endocarditis. Emerg Med Clin North Am 2018;36(4): 645–63.

46. Crawford MH, Durack DT. Clinical presentation of infective endocarditis. Cardiol Clin 2003;21(2):159–66, v.

47. Steckelberg JM, Wilson WR. Risk factors for infective endocarditis. Infect Dis Clin North Am 1993;7(1):9–19.

48. Wu Z, Chen Y, Xiao T, et al. Epidemiology and risk factors of infective endocarditis in a tertiary hospital in China from 2007 to 2016. BMC Infect Dis 2020;20(1):428.

49. Durack DT, Lukes AS, Bright DK. New criteria for diagnosis of infective endocarditis: utilization of specific echocardiographic findings. Duke Endocarditis Serv Am J Med 1994;96(3):200–9.

50. Lee CH, Tsai WC, Liu PY, et al. Epidemiologic features of infective endocarditis in Taiwanese adults involving native valves. Am J Cardiol 2007;100(8):1282–5.

51. Joseph JP, Meddows TR, Webster DP, et al. Prioritizing echocardiography in Staphylococcus aureus bacteraemia. J Antimicrob Chemother 2013;68(2):444–9.

52. Mostaghim AS, Lo HYA, Khardori N. A retrospective epidemiologic study to define risk factors, microbiology, and clinical outcomes of infective endocarditis in a large tertiary-care teaching hospital. SAGE Open Med 2017;5. 2050312117741772.

53. Thuny F, Fournier PE, Casalta JP, et al. Investigation of blood culture-negative early prosthetic valve endocarditis reveals high prevalence of fungi. Heart 2010;96(10):743–7.

54. Asopa S, Patel A, Khan OA, et al. Non-bacterial thrombotic endocarditis. Eur J Cardiothorac Surg 2007;32(5):696–701.

55. Fournier PE, Thuny F, Richet H, et al. Comprehensive diagnostic strategy for blood culture-negative endocarditis: a prospective study of 819 new cases. Clin Infect Dis 2010;51(2):131–40.

56. Sivak JA, Vora AN, Navar AM, et al. An Approach to Improve the Negative Predictive Value and Clinical Utility of Transthoracic Echocardiography in Suspected Native Valve Infective Endocarditis. J Am Soc Echocardiogr 2016;29(4):315–22.

57. Reynolds HR, Jagen MA, Tunick PA, et al. Sensitivity of transthoracic versus transesophageal echocardiography for the detection of native valve vegetations in the modern era. J Am Soc Echocardiogr 2003;16(1):67–70.

58. Galiana A, Coy J, Gimeno A, et al. Evaluation of the sepsis flow chip assay for the diagnosis of blood infections. PLoS One 2017;12(5):e0177627.

59. Rothman RE, Majmudar MD, Kelen GD, et al. Detection of bacteremia in emergency department patients at risk for infective endocarditis using universal 16S rRNA primers in a decontaminated polymerase chain reaction assay. J Infect Dis 2002;186(11):1677–81.

60. Samuel LP, Tibbetts RJ, Agotesku A, et al. Evaluation of a microarray-based assay for rapid identification of Gram-positive organisms and resistance markers in positive blood cultures. J Clin Microbiol 2013;51(4):1188–92.

61. Rossi SE, Goodman PC, Franquet T. Nonthrombotic pulmonary emboli. AJR Am J Roentgenol 2000;174(6):1499–508.

62. Li JS, Sexton DJ, Mick N, et al. Proposed modifications to the Duke criteria for the diagnosis of infective endocarditis. Clin Infect Dis 2000;30(4):633–8.

63. Prendergast BD, Tornos P. Surgery for infective endocarditis: who and when? Circulation 2010;121(9):1141–52.

64. Gilbert DN, Chambers HF, Eliopoulos GM, et al. The Sanford guide to antimicrobial therapy. 50th edition. Antimicrobial Therapy; 2019.

65. Fowler VG Jr, Boucher HW, Corey GR, et al. Daptomycin versus standard therapy for bacteremia and endocarditis caused by Staphylococcus aureus. N Engl J Med 2006;355(7):653–65.

66. Iversen K, Ihlemann N, Gill SU, et al. Partial oral versus intravenous antibiotic treatment of endocarditis. N Engl J Med 2019;380(5):415–24.

67. Heiro M, Helenius H, Hurme S, et al. Long-term outcome of infective endocarditis: a study on patients surviving over one year after the initial episode treated in a Finnish teaching hospital during 25 years. BMC Infect Dis 2008;8:49.

68. Martinez-Selles M, Munoz P, Estevez A, et al. Long-term outcome of infective endocarditis in non-intravenous drug users. Mayo Clin Proc 2008;83(11):1213–7.

69. Thuny F, Giorgi R, Habachi R, et al. Excess mortality and morbidity in patients surviving infective endocarditis. Am Heart J 2012;164(1):94–101.

70. Duval X, Leport C. Prophylaxis of infective endocarditis: current tendencies, continuing controversies. Lancet Infect Dis 2008;8(4):225–32.

71. Lockhart PB. Guidelines for prevention of infective endocarditis: an explanation of the changes. J Am Dent Assoc 2008;139(Suppl):2S.

High Sensitivity Troponins

Tyler Thomas Hempel, MD, Amy Wyatt, DO*

KEYWORDS

- High-sensitivity troponin • Chest pain • Cardiac biomarkers • Emergency medicine
- Acute coronary syndrome • Cardiac rule out • Myocardial infarction • Acute MI

KEY POINTS

- High-sensitivity cardiac troponin assays (hs-cTn) are the recommended cardiac biomarkers in all major US and European guidelines.
- The hs-cTn assays can detect circulating troponin levels down to 1 ng/L, 10–100 times lower than conventional troponin assays.
- When used in the appropriate clinical context, the hs-cTn assays allow the rapid rule out of non-ST-elevation myocardial infarction, resulting in decreased emergency department lengths of stay, decreased observation hospitalizations, less cardiac testing, and lower health care costs, while maintaining safety.
- There are many proposed diagnostic pathways and experts recommend that each institution choose a single pathway for consistent use by all providers.

CLINICAL VIGNETTE

A 55-year-old man with a history of peptic ulcer, hypertension, and hyperlipidemia presents to the emergency department (ED) with acute onset of chest pain that began 4 hours before arrival. The pain is worse with exertion and eating, radiates into his left arm, and is associated with nausea. An electrocardiogram (ECG) obtained during triage shows nonspecific T-wave inversions. No prior ECGs are available for comparison. The patient appears well and is in no acute distress. Vital signs are normal, and the physical examination is unremarkable. As a seasoned clinician, you are concerned about acute coronary syndrome (ACS). You develop a plan to obtain basic laboratory studies, chest radiograph, and troponin. The results are unremarkable. Based on your clinical gestalt and the HEART score, you determine that the patient has a moderate probability of a major adverse cardiac event (MACE) in the next month. You plan to transfer him to the observation unit for further evaluation and management. However, given the overcrowded and understaffed hospital, you wonder if this patient would be safe to discharge. In preparation for an ED operations meeting, you have been reading

Department of Emergency Medicine, UPMC Harrisburg, 205 South Front Street, Brady 3 Suite 3A, Harrisburg, PA 17104, USA
* Corresponding author.
E-mail address: Wyattal@upmc.edu

Emerg Med Clin N Am 40 (2022) 809–821
https://doi.org/10.1016/j.emc.2022.07.002
0733-8627/22/© 2022 Elsevier Inc. All rights reserved.

about high-sensitivity troponin and ask yourself whether this new test could expedite patient care in a safe and efficient manner.

INTRODUCTION

In 2018, chest pain accounted for over 7 million ED visits in the United States, nearly 5% of all ED patient complaints.[1] Despite the expertise of the emergency medicine (EM) physician in assessing patients for life-threatening conditions, ACS is among the most difficult conditions to rapidly and reliably diagnose given the diversity in presentation and the paucity of associated physical examination findings.[2,3] Given these obstacles, EM physicians rely on additional diagnostic testing, in particular cardiac biomarkers. The most recent advancement in cardiac testing is the fifth generation of high-sensitivity cardiac troponin (hs-cTn) assays.[4] In this article, we review the history of cardiac biomarkers, the role of hs-cTn in diagnostic pathways and current guidelines, limitations of hs-cTn use and interpretation, and, finally, future applications of these assays.

THE HISTORY OF BIOMARKERS AND TROPONIN TESTING

For over 50 years, scientists have tried to identify a biomarker to aid in the diagnosis of ACS and acute myocardial infarction (AMI).[5] To understand the evolution and progress made in this field, it is important to explore the ultimate goal of this endeavor. Numerous panels have debated the characteristics that make an ideal marker (**Fig. 1**).

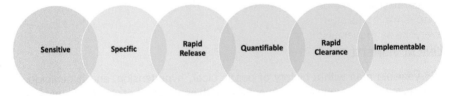

Fig. 1. Characteristics of an ideal biomarker.

Some common characteristics deemed important include the following:[5–7]

- High sensitivity (ie, able to detect even a minimal amount of damage to the heart)
- High specificity for cardiac damage (ie, damage to noncardiac tissue should not cause false positives)
- Rapid release from cardiac tissue (ie, present in serum shortly after AMI)
- Rapid measurability (ie, laboratory turnaround time is quick)
- Quantifiable (ie, able to delineate severity of infarct)
- Rapid clearance (ie, able to determine the trajectory of a patient's clinical course)
- Implementability (ie, cheap, quick, and easy to measure)

While the perfect biomarker does not currently exist, there have been great advances over the years (**Fig. 2**).[4] A brief summary of the history of cardiac biomarkers is included for context, with a focus on troponin testing and characteristics of the fifth-generation hs-cTn, which has become more popular over the past decade.[8,9]

1954 and the Creation of the First Biomarker

The first cardiac biomarker, developed in 1954, was serum glutamic oxaloacetic transaminase, now referred to as aspartate aminotransferase (AST).[5] AST elevation has

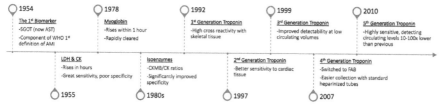

Fig. 2. Timeline of cardiac biomarker advances: 1954–2022.

high sensitivity (up to 90%) but low specificity, as it is also present in hepatocytes.[10] It was used routinely in the 1960s and was a component of the World Health Organization's definition of AMI in their first report on the classification of heart disease.[4]

The Second-Generation Biomarkers

Tests for lactate dehydrogenase (LDH) and creatinine kinase (CK) were developed in 1955 and both were noted to rise acutely within hours of the onset of an AMI. Both tests were found to be highly sensitive (98%), however, they suffered from a lack of specificity as LDH is also found in skeletal muscle, liver tissue, and erythrocytes, and CK can be found in the brain and skeletal muscles.[5]

The Promise of Myoglobin

In 1978, scientists developed a serum test for myoglobin, and by 1986, a rapid test enabled clinical use. Myoglobin can be detected in blood as early as 1 hour after myocardial injury and peaks at 4 to 7 hours. Given its ability to rapidly detect changes in ischemia, it was often used to determine the success of thrombolysis for AMI. However, like its predecessors, myoglobin suffered from a lack of specificity as it is also found in skeletal muscle.[5]

The Development of Isoenzymes

In the late 1970s and early 1980s, advancements in laboratory techniques allowed scientists to isolate cardiac-specific isoenzymes, most importantly CK myocardial band (CK-MB).[5] CK-MB to CK ratios become altered 4 to 9 hours after AMI[6] and were found to have specificity and sensitivity greater than 90%.[7] These favorable test characteristics allowed CK ratios to be used clinically for over two decades.[4,5]

The Age of Troponin

In 1963, Professor Setsuro Ebashi identified a protein in the cardiac myocyte that binds calcium and helps activate the myosin–actin complex. It is this protein that would eventually be known as troponin.[5] In the early 1970s, it was discovered troponin has three separate components:

1. Troponin C (TnC): binding site for calcium ion
2. Troponin I (TnI): inhibits (in absence of calcium) adenosine triphospatase activity
3. Troponin T (TnT): binding site for tropomyosin

Over the next few decades of study, it was noted that TnC is also found in skeletal tissue; however, TnI and TnT are highly specific for cardiac tissue and became known as cardiac troponins (cTn).[4,5]

In the 1980s, scientists began to examine the utility of cTn as a cardiac biomarker, but initial tests took 2 days to result.

In 1992, the automatization of first-generation immunoassay troponins drastically improved test turnaround time; however, they suffered from high cross-reactivity with skeletal tissue. In 1997, second-generation troponins with more sensitivity for cardiac tissue were created and by 1999 third-generation tests had improved upon detectability at low circulating volumes. In 2007, fourth-generation troponins switched to fragment antigen-binding,[5] and the collection was made easier with the ability to use standard heparinized tubes.[11]

Fifth-Generation High-Sensitivity Troponin

Fifth-generation troponin assays were first introduced into clinical use in 2010 and represent a significant improvement in sensitivity over the prior generation.[12] These hs-cTn assays are now able to detect circulating levels down to 1 ng/L, 10–100 times lower than prior generations.[4] A substantial amount of information on the clinical utility of this test has been gained over the last decade.[3,4,13–15]

Many parts of the world began utilizing hs-cTn assays shortly after their development, and the number of assays available worldwide has grown substantially since that time. In contrast, there are only three hs-cTn assays available in the United States, with the first receiving the Food and Drug Administration's approval in 2017.

When using hs-cTn assays, there are several important terms clinicians must understand:[3,8,13,14]

- Limit of detection (LoD): This is defined as the lowest possible amount of circulating troponin that an assay can detect in 95% of samples.
- The 99th percentile of a normal reference population (99th percentile): If the circulating troponin level was tested in a healthy asymptomatic population, then 99% of individuals would have a level below this value.
- Delta value (delta): This is the difference between two hs-cTn levels that are drawn over a period in the same patient.

It is important to understand that these values vary between the different commercially available assays; therefore, a strict numerical comparison is complicated.[3,8,13,14] There have been efforts to create tools to assist in the comparison of these details, such as the compass-MI project, which provides an online calculator.[16]

One of the hopes for hs-cTn was to rapidly rule out a non-ST-elevation myocardial infarction (NSTEMI), preferably with a single laboratory draw.[4,8,15,17–19] Initial studies showed that a single hs-cTn below the 99th percentile was not sensitive enough (90%), although it did have a relatively good specificity (>70%). Further studies demonstrated that decreasing the cutoff to the LoD substantially improved sensitivity to nearly 99% but sacrificed specificity.[20]

To optimize the clinical application of hs-cTn, rapid diagnostic protocols incorporating the LoD, the 99th percentile, and delta have been developed. These protocols attempt to maximize sensitivity and negative predictive value (NPV), increase specificity, and facilitate rapid and cost-effective care.[3,8,9,19,21,22]

While hs-cTn can be beneficial in the appropriate clinical setting, it is not meant to be used alone. A clinician must still rely on the mainstays of patient evaluation including history, physical examination, and interpretation of ECG(s).[13,14,18]

RAPID DIAGNOSTIC PROTOCOLS

There have been numerous studies looking at how hs-cTn can be used to rapidly rule out NSTEMI with high sensitivity. Multiple protocols have been created that typically follow a consistent pattern (**Fig. 3**):

- Patients with a history that is concerning for ACS, without STEMI, are identified.
- An initial troponin is obtained on arrival; ie, 0-hour hs-cTn.

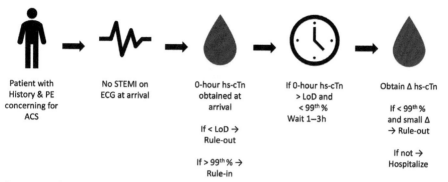

Fig. 3. Rapid diagnostic protocol. This image represents an example of the pattern typical of hs-cTn rapid diagnostic protocols found in literature and institutions.

- If the 0-hour hs-cTn is below the LoD, then patients are ruled out for NSTEMI.
- If the 0-hour hs-cTn is above the 99th percentile, then these patients rule-in.
- If the 0-hour hs-cTn is above the LoD and below the 99th percentile, then a repeat hs-cTn is drawn at a predetermined interval (eg, 1 to 3 hours) after the initial blood draw.
- If the second hs-cTn is below both the 99th percentile and a prespecified delta, patients are ruled out for NSTEMI. Otherwise, the patient is kept for hospitalization.

Protocols often have a caveat that the onset of chest pain just before arrival (typically 1 to 3 hours) cannot be ruled out with only a 0-hour hs-cTn.

0/1-Hour Troponin Protocols

The European Society of Cardiology (ESC) first published a 0/1-hour hs-cTn protocol in 2015.[23] In their most recent 2020 guidelines, this is their preferred testing strategy. This new guideline recommendation is based on a robust body of data accumulated over the past decade.[14]

The RAPID-TnT (Rapid Assessment of Possible Acute Coronary Syndrome in the Emergency Department with High-Sensitivity Troponin T) study from Australia is one of the largest prospective trials evaluating the 0/1-hour protocol. It assessed whether a 0/1-hour hs-cTn protocol was noninferior to a traditional 0/3-hour protocol.

They enrolled over 3000 patients between 2015 and 2019 and randomly assigned them to either a 0/1-hour arm or a 0/3-hour arm. Of note, they used hs-cTn assays in both arms, but the 0/3-hour arm utilized cutoffs for conventional troponins, substantially higher than the hs-cTn 99th percentile cutoff.

The primary endpoints of all-cause mortality and AMI at 30-days were approximately 1% in both arms. The secondary endpoints demonstrated significant benefit to the 0/1-hour arm. This included decreasing length of stay by approximately 90 minutes, and increasing ED discharges by approximately 13%. This led the authors of the article to conclude that a 0/1-hour protocol using hs-cTn was noninferior to standard practice and "enabled more rapid discharge of patients with the suspected acute coronary syndrome."[24]

0/2-Hour Troponin Protocols

Some clinicians worry that because of the physiologic time it takes for troponin to leak into the bloodstream a 0/1-hour protocol may miss some NSTEMIs and have therefore proposed a 0/2-hour protocol to increase sensitivity. A 0/2-hour protocol has been studied, and while the evidence is less robust, it is still a recommended algorithm per the ESC 2020 guidelines.[14]

The APACE (Advantageous Predictors of Acute Coronary Syndrome Evaluation) study is an international multicenter study coordinated by The University Hospital Basel in Switzerland. They have published numerous studies on hs-cTn. One of their studies with 1148 patients derived a 0/2-hour protocol that maximized sensitivity and NPV, and a subsequent study validated the protocol.[23]

In the validation study, they were able to safely risk-stratify patients with possible ACS. The stratification groups included the following:

- A "rule-out" group
  - These patients were discharged after initial evaluation
    - 78% of study population
    - 100% survival rate at 1 year
    - AMI rate <1% at 30 days
- An "observational zone" group
  - These patients were admitted for observation
    - 14% of study population
    - 96% survival rate at 1 year
    - AMI rate of approximately 15% at 30 days
- A "rule-in" group
  - These patients were admitted with the diagnosis of AMI
    - 8% of study population
    - 87.5% survival rate at 1 year
    - AMI rate of 77.5% at 30 days
      - Some rule-in patients had elevated hs-cTn that were ultimately related to other causes, including pericarditis, congestive heart failure, or stable CAD.

0/3-Hour Troponin Protocols

The ESC 2015 guidelines recommended a 0/3-hour protocol in which clinicians first calculate a GRACE score,[25] although newer data show that 0/3-hour protocols without a scoring tool may be safe.[26] In the original ESC protocol, if all the listed criteria are met, then the patient can be ruled out:

- Chest pain onset >6 hours
- Patient is pain-free
- GRACE score <140
- 0-hour hs-cTn < 99th percentile

If the chest pain onset is < 6 hours, then a patient can be ruled out if a 3-hour hs-cTn is:

- Still <99th percentile AND
- The delta < prespecified value

All patients who do not meet those criteria require further evaluation.[25]

Wildi and colleagues[27] demonstrated the safety of this protocol in a prospective international multicenter study published in 2016 that enrolled over 2700 patients. They found:

- Patients with onset > 6 hours and a single negative hs-cTn
  - 99.6% ruled out correctly
- Patients with onset < 6 hours and two negative hs-cTn
  - 99. 5% ruled out correctly
- Specificity ranged between 40% and 50% depending on the hs-cTn assay used
- Secondary endpoint of mortality rate at 3 months was 0% for all groups

While the 2020 ESC guidelines state a 0/3-hour protocol should be "considered," they also note several recent large studies suggest it "balances efficacy and safety less well" than other protocols.[14]

Rapid Diagnostic Protocols + Scoring Tools

Some clinicians raise concern over low specificity with traditional hs-cTn protocols, potentially resulting in increased admissions.[4,9,18,28,29] Others raise concern that traditional hs-cTn protocols are designed to rule patients in or out for AMI, not to rule out other causes of 30-day MACE or to determine which patients are suitable for discharge.[2,3,17,18,30–32] As a result, pathways that add a scoring tool, such as HEART or ED-ACS, to the original hs-cTn protocols have been proposed. In these combined pathways, clinicians first apply a scoring tool to stratify patients into risk categories. The original protocol is then followed, however, different hs-cTn thresholds are applied based on the patient's risk. These higher thresholds result in an increased number of patients able to be discharged after a single troponin while maintaining high sensitivity and NPV.[2,33]

Nilsson and colleagues performed a secondary analysis of data from a prospective observational study that included 939 patients. This aimed to evaluate the combination of either the HEART score or the ED-ACS score with the ESC 0/1-hour protocol on rates of 30-day MACE, including unstable angina. They found that, in addition to maintaining good sensitivity and improving NPV for 30-day MACE, the addition of either risk score increased the number of patients potentially safe for discharge from 30% to 50%.[2]

This remains an area of controversy, with questions regarding the tradeoff between increasing complexity of use and potential impacts on safety.[19,21,22,30,31]

GUIDELINES

The major organizations in the United States and Europe have released updated guidelines to assist with the evaluation, diagnosis, and management of patients with the suspected ACS. In 2020, the ESC released its updated guidelines.[14] In 2021, the American Heart Association (AHA), in conjunction with the American College of Cardiology (ACC), the American Society of Echocardiography (ASE), CHEST, the Society for Academic Emergency Medicine (SAEM), the Society of Cardiovascular Computed Tomography (SCCT), and the Society for Cardiovascular Magnetic Resonance (SCMR) released their guidelines.[13] These guidelines universally recommend the use of hs-cTn over conventional troponin due to the following reasons:

- High diagnostic accuracy at low cost
- High NPV
- High sensitivity
- High specificity to cardiac tissue
- Rapid detectability after onset of symptoms (usually within 1 hour)

We now discuss the highest yield points relating to biomarkers from these extensive guidelines.

2020 European Society of Cardiology Guidelines for the Management of Acute Coronary Syndrome in Patients Presenting without Persistent ST-Segment Elevation

- The addition of hs-cTn resulted in ~4% relative and ~20% absolute increase in the diagnosis of AMI, correctly reclassifying patients previously diagnosed with unstable angina.[14]
- Most rule-in patients with a diagnosis other than AMI still had diagnoses requiring invasive coronary angiography.
- The use of specific protocols is recommended:
  - 0/1-hour protocol = Best option
  - 0/2-hour protocol = Second best option
  - 0/3-hour protocol = Alternative option, however, most recent data favors the 0/1 or 0/2 protocols
- There are several caveats for the recommended protocols.
  - Protocols should always be used in conjunction with all other clinical information.
  - The 0/1- and 0/2-hour protocols apply irrespective of time of symptom onset.
    - There is high safety and sensitivity even in the subgroup of patients presenting with symptom onset less than 2 hours.
    - There are insufficient data at this time for those with symptom onset less than 1 hour, thus obtaining a 3-hour troponin should be considered in this population.
  - Late troponin increases have been described in ~1% of patients, so if clinical suspicion is very high, or with recurrent chest pain, consider serial troponins.
- Troponin T and I are comparable for diagnostic accuracy.
- Serial troponins should be obtained for risk stratification in patients with established AMI, as a higher level equates to a higher risk of death.

American Heart Association/American College of Cardiology, American Society of Echocardiography, CHEST, Society for Academic Emergency Medicine, Society of Cardiovascular Computed Tomography, and Society for Cardiovascular Magnetic Resonance 2021 Guidelines for the Evaluation and Diagnosis of Chest Pain

- Each hs-cTn assay has its own specific criteria (ie, LoD, 99th percentile, and so on); so, it is important to be familiar with the particular assay being used.[13]
- All patients should be risk stratified into low, moderate, or high risk for ACS and risk of 30-day MACE.
  - Multiple suggested clinical decision pathways are provided, with no specific preference.
    - It is, however, strongly recommended that every institution implement a *single* pathway.
  - Unlike conventional troponin, hs-cTn does not require the use of a risk score because it may be more predictive than other clinical components.
  - A pathway that utilizes a 0-hour troponin and a second troponin 1 to 3 hours after the first is recommended, but there is no position on the best option.
- Myocardial injury can be excluded if all of the following criteria are met:
  - Symptoms of ACS for >3 hours
  - Normal ECG
  - 0-hour hs-cTn < LoD
- Elevations in hs-cTn in the setting of chest pain are associated with a higher risk of adverse outcomes regardless of the cause.

LIMITATIONS

First, it is important to understand that evaluating the literature is complicated by multiple factors, including a change from the third to fourth universal definition of acute MI, the considerable number of different assays available with their individual cutoffs, the variation in the use of either sex-specific or universal cutoffs, exclusion criteria, and a difference in primary endpoints between diagnosis of index AMI versus the risk of 30-day MACE.

Also, there are several clinical variables whose impacts on hs-cTn remain controversial.[13,14,18,34]

Universal Versus Sex-Specific Cutoffs

There is clear evidence that healthy women have a lower level of circulating troponin than men and therefore a lower 99th percentile upper limit of normal.[3,9,18] Questions remain as to whether the difference is clinically significant, and there is concern that sex-specific cutoffs might add too much confusion and hamper protocol implementation.[3,8,22,29] Currently the ESC 2020 guidelines recommend universal cutoffs[14] while both the 2018 task force on the universal definition of AMI and the 2021 AHA guidelines recommend sex-specific cutoffs.[13,34]

Age-Specific Cutoffs

Concentrations of circulating levels of troponin increase with age regardless of comorbidities, and it has been proposed that thresholds should change with age as well.[18] There are currently no age-specific guidelines.

Time of Onset of Symptoms

While it is well established that symptom onset >3 hours before evaluation is sufficient to detect circulating hs-cTn if there has been a myocardial injury, controversy remains for patients presenting <3 hours.[3,8,13,14,22] There is currently limited data to support detectability in patients with earlier symptom onset.[2,15,35] There is evidence that the addition of a scoring tool to a rapid diagnostic protocol may be safe for symptom onset <3 hours.[8,22]

Impact of Renal Disease

Patients with underlying renal disease often have detectable circulating troponin, but the causative mechanism is still unclear. Studies have demonstrated that a negative hs-cTn maintains sensitivity and NPV for rule out. Levels above the 99th percentile have a poor prognosis regardless of cause but worse specificity and PPV for rule in. A rising or falling delta level remains diagnostic, so serial levels are important in this patient population.[3,4,8,30,36,37]

FUTURE AREAS OF INTEREST

The world of cardiac biomarkers continues to evolve. Point-of-care testing is just becoming available for hs-cTns and will require evaluation for safety and real-world impact. In theory, it could enable more rapid dispositions, especially in those individuals who rule in or rule out with a 0-hour troponin.[14,18]

Also uncertain is the role of hs-cTn outside of the evaluation of ACS. The 2021 ACC guidelines make clear that the "presence of myocardial injury in the setting of chest pain, regardless of cause, is associated with a higher risk of adverse outcomes."[13] While it makes sense that myocardial injury in any setting is a concerning finding, there are still a lot of questions to be answered about real-world impacts.[4,13,14] Will this change the identification and management of right heart strain for pulmonary embolism? Will hypertensive urgency patients actually be hypertensive emergencies? Can the presence or absence of hs-cTn help to determine when a disease process is clinically significant and requires further evaluation and treatment?

Less important to the EM physician, but still of future interest, are applications, such as monitoring cardiotoxic effects of certain medications, monitoring chronic cardiac or renal disease, screening for risk stratification of future cardiac disease, and measuring changes after exercise stress testing, and the impacts of extreme exercise.[5,8,13,14]

VIGNETTE CONCLUSION

During your time off you read up on hs-cTn. You realize that because your patient's symptoms had been going on for 4 hours, a hs-cTn below the LoD would have ruled out NSTEMI with 99% sensitivity. Even if his hs-cTn was above the LoD but below the 99th percentile, a repeat hs-cTn at 1, 2, or 3 hours without a significant rise also would have adequately ruled out NSTEMI. Your hospital system has good outpatient resources and cardiology follow-up, and you determine that adding hs-cTn to your testing system has the potential to decrease both ED lengths of stay and hospitalizations. You plan to present this information to the operations committee as a novel way to improve workflow and decrease the hospital burden in these trying times.

CLINICS CARE POINTS

- Be familiar with the care pathway/guidelines at your institution, as cutoff levels will be dependent upon the timing of laboratory draws.
- Patients presenting rapidly after the onset of symptoms should have a delta troponin.
- Most patients will have a detectable high-sensitivity cardiac troponin (hs-cTn). Thinking should shift from "positive" or "negative" and focus instead on absolute numbers and trends as these have prognostic value.
- Troponin levels change rapidly; so trends are easily detectable over short periods.
- Elevations in hs-cTn correspond to myocardial injury but not necessarily myocardial infarction, so be certain to consider other causes.
- The higher the absolute hs-cTn level, the greater the positive predictive value for acute myocardial infarction.
- Elevations in hs-cTn in the setting of chest pain are associated with a higher risk of adverse outcomes regardless of cause and should be concerning.
- Renal failure patients with undetectable or low levels are valid, but elevated levels are more difficult to interpret and may benefit from trending.

DISCLOSURE

The authors have nothing to disclose.

REFERENCES

1. Cairns C, Kang K, Santo L. National hospital ambulatory medical care survey: 2018 emergency department summary tables. National Center for Health Statistics. Available at: https://www.cdc.gov/nchs/data/nhamcs/web_tables/2018-ed-web-tables-508.pdf. Accessed January 24, 2022.

2. Nilsson T, Johannesson E, Lundager Forberg J, et al. Diagnostic accuracy of the HEART pathway and EDACS-ADP when combined with a 0-hour/1-hour hs-cTnT protocol for assessment of acute chest pain patients. Emerg Med J 2021;38(11): 808–13.
3. Twerenbold R, Boeddinghaus J, Nestelberger T, et al. Clinical use of high-sensitivity cardiac troponin in patients with suspected myocardial infarction. J Am Coll Cardiol 2017;70(8):996–1012.
4. Garg P, Morris P, Fazlanie AL, et al. Cardiac biomarkers of acute coronary syndrome: from history to high-sensitivity cardiac troponin. Intern Emerg Med 2017;12(2):147–55.
5. Danese E, Montagnana M. An historical approach to the diagnostic biomarkers of acute coronary syndrome. Ann Transl Med 2016;4(10):194.
6. Mythili S, Malathi N. Diagnostic markers of acute myocardial infarction. Biomed Rep 2015;3(6):743–8.
7. Aydin S, Ugur K, Aydin S, et al. Biomarkers in acute myocardial infarction: current perspectives. Vasc Health Risk Manag 2019;15:1–10.
8. Januzzi JL Jr, Mahler SA, Christenson RH, et al. Recommendations for institutions transitioning to high-sensitivity troponin testing: JACC Scientific Expert Panel. J Am Coll Cardiol 2019;73(9):1059–77.
9. Anand A, Shah ASV, Beshiri A, et al. Global adoption of high-sensitivity cardiac troponins and the universal definition of myocardial infarction. Clin Chem 2019; 65(3):484–9.
10. Johnston CC, Bolton EC. Cardiac enzymes. Ann Emerg Med 1982;11(1):27–35.
11. Hermsen D, Apple F, Garcia-Beltràn L, et al. Results from a multicenter evaluation of the 4th generation Elecsys Troponin T assay. Clin Lab 2007;53(1–2):1–9.
12. Chapman AR, Mills NL. High-sensitivity cardiac troponin and the early rule out of myocardial infarction: time for action. Heart 2020;106(13):955–7.
13. Gulati M, Levy PD, Mukherjee D, et al. 2021 AHA/ACC/ASE/CHEST/SAEM/SCCT/ SCMR guideline for the evaluation and diagnosis of chest pain: a report of the american college of cardiology/american heart association joint committee on clinical practice guidelines. Circulation 2021;144(22):e368–454 [published correction appears in Circulation. 2021 Nov 30;144(22):e455].
14. Collet JP, Thiele H, Barbato E, et al. 2020 ESC Guidelines for the management of acute coronary syndromes in patients presenting without persistent ST-segment elevation. Eur Heart J 2021;42(14):1289–367 [published correction appears in Eur Heart J. 2021 May 14;42(19):1908] [published correction appears in Eur Heart J. 2021 May 14;42(19):1925] [published correction appears in Eur Heart J. 2021 May 13;:].
15. Pickering JW, Than MP, Cullen L, et al. Rapid rule-out of acute myocardial infarction with a single high-sensitivity cardiac troponin T measurement below the limit of detection: a collaborative meta-analysis. Ann Intern Med 2017;166(10):715–24 [published correction appears in Ann Intern Med. 2017 Oct 3;167(7):528].
16. Neumann JT, Twerenbold R, Ojeda F, et al. Application of high-sensitivity troponin in suspected myocardial infarction. N Engl J Med 2019;380(26):2529–40.
17. Cook B, McCord J, Hudson M, et al. Baseline high sensitivity cardiac troponin I level below limit of quantitation rules out acute myocardial infarction in the emergency department. Crit Pathw Cardiol 2021;20(1):4–9.
18. Giannitsis E, Blankenberg S, Christenson RH, et al. Critical appraisal of the 2020 ESC guideline recommendations on diagnosis and risk assessment in patients with suspected non-ST-segment elevation acute coronary syndrome. Clin Res Cardiol 2021;110(9):1353–68.

19. Carlton E. Do cardiac risk scores only muddy the waters? Emerg Med J 2021; 38(11):806–7.
20. Zhelev Z, Hyde C, Youngman E, et al. Diagnostic accuracy of single baseline measurement of Elecsys troponin T high-sensitive assay for diagnosis of acute myocardial infarction in emergency department: systematic review and meta-analysis. BMJ 2015;350:h15.
21. Mueller C, Boeddinghaus J, Nestelberger T. Downstream consequences of implementing high-sensitivity cardiac troponin: why indication and education matter. J Am Coll Cardiol 2021;77(25):3180–3.
22. Twerenbold R, Costabel JP, Nestelberger T, et al. Outcome of applying the ESC 0/1-hour algorithm in patients with suspected myocardial infarction. J Am Coll Cardiol 2019;74(4):483–94.
23. Reichlin T, Cullen L, Parsonage WA, et al. Two-hour algorithm for triage toward rule-out and rule-in of acute myocardial infarction using high-sensitivity cardiac troponin T. Am J Med 2015;128(4):369–79.e4.
24. Chew DP, Lambrakis K, Blyth A, et al. A randomized trial of a 1-hour troponin T protocol in suspected acute coronary syndromes: the rapid assessment of possible acute coronary syndrome in the emergency department with high-sensitivity troponin T study (RAPID-TnT). Circulation 2019;140(19):1543–56 [published correction appears in Circulation. 2021 Jun 22;143(25):e1118].
25. Roffi M, Patrono C, Collet JP, et al. 2015 ESC Guidelines for the management of acute coronary syndromes in patients presenting without persistent ST-segment elevation: task force for the management of acute coronary syndromes in patients presenting without persistent ST-segment elevation of the european society of cardiology (ESC). Eur Heart J 2016;37(3):267–315.
26. Badertscher P, Boeddinghaus J, Twerenbold R, et al. Direct comparison of the 0/1h and 0/3h algorithms for early rule-out of acute myocardial infarction. Circulation 2018;137(23):2536–8.
27. Wildi K, Nelles B, Twerenbold R, et al. Safety and efficacy of the 0 h/3 h protocol for rapid rule out of myocardial infarction. Am Heart J 2016;181:16–25.
28. Twerenbold R, Jaeger C, Rubini Gimenez M, et al. Impact of high-sensitivity cardiac troponin on use of coronary angiography, cardiac stress testing, and time to discharge in suspected acute myocardial infarction. Eur Heart J 2016;37(44): 3324–32.
29. Vasile VC, Jaffe AS. High-sensitivity cardiac troponin in the evaluation of possible AMI: Expert analysis. Am Coll Cardiol 2018. Available at: https://www.acc.org/latest-in-cardiology/articles/2018/07/16/09/17/high-sensitivity-cardiac-troponin-in-the-evaluation-of-possible-ami. July 16. Accessed January 24, 2022.
30. Wildi K, Cullen L, Twerenbold R, et al. Direct comparison of 2 rule-out strategies for acute myocardial infarction: 2-h accelerated diagnostic protocol vs 2-h algorithm. Clin Chem 2017;63(7):1227–36. https://doi.org/10.1373/clinchem.2016. 268359.
31. Chiang CH, Chiang CH, Pickering JW, et al. Performance of the European Society of Cardiology 0/1-Hour, 0/2-Hour, and 0/3-Hour algorithms for rapid triage of acute myocardial Infarction: an international collaborative meta-analysis. Ann Intern Med 2022;175(1):101–13.
32. Pickering JW, Greenslade JH, Cullen L, et al. Assessment of the European Society of Cardiology 0-Hour/1-Hour algorithm to rule-out and rule-in acute myocardial infarction. Circulation 2016;134(20):1532–41.
33. Greenslade JH, Carlton EW, Van Hise C, et al. Diagnostic accuracy of a new high-sensitivity troponin I assay and five accelerated diagnostic pathways for ruling

out acute myocardial infarction and acute coronary syndrome. Ann Emerg Med 2018;71(4):439–51.e3.

34. Thygesen K, Alpert JS, Jaffe AS, et al. Fourth universal definition of myocardial infarction (2018). Eur Heart J 2019;40(3):237–69.

35. Carlton E, Campbell S, Ingram J, et al. Randomised controlled trial of the Limit of Detection of Troponin and ECG Discharge (LoDED) strategy versus usual care in adult patients with chest pain attending the emergency department: study protocol. BMJ Open 2018;8(10):e025339.

36. Twerenbold R, Badertscher P, Boeddinghaus J, et al. 0/1-hour triage algorithm for myocardial infarction in patients with renal dysfunction. Circulation 2018;137(5):436–51.

37. Miller-Hodges E, Anand A, Shah ASV, et al. High-sensitivity cardiac troponin and the risk stratification of patients with renal impairment presenting with suspected acute coronary syndrome. Circulation 2018;137(5):425–35.

UNITED STATES POSTAL SERVICE®

Statement of Ownership, Management, and Circulation
(All Periodicals Publications Except Requester Publications)

1. Publication Title
EMERGENCY MEDICINE CLINICS OF NORTH AMERICA

2. Publication Number
000 – 714

3. Filing Date
9/18/2022

4. Issue Frequency
FEB, MAY, AUG, NOV

5. Number of Issues Published Annually
4

6. Annual Subscription Price
$370.00

7. Complete Mailing Address of Known Office of Publication *(Not printer)* *(Street, city, county, state, and ZIP+4®)*
ELSEVIER INC.
230 Park Avenue, Suite 800
New York, NY 10169

Contact Person
Malathi Samayan

Telephone *(Include area code)*
91-44-4299-4507

8. Complete Mailing Address of Headquarters or General Business Office of Publisher *(Not printer)*
ELSEVIER INC.
230 Park Avenue, Suite 800
New York, NY 10169

9. Full Names and Complete Mailing Addresses of Publisher, Editor, and Managing Editor *(Do not leave blank)*

Publisher *(Name and complete mailing address)*
Dolores Meloni, ELSEVIER INC.
1600 JOHN F KENNEDY BLVD. SUITE 1800
PHILADELPHIA, PA 19103-2899

Editor *(Name and complete mailing address)*
JOANNA COLLETT, ELSEVIER INC.
1600 JOHN F KENNEDY BLVD. SUITE 1800
PHILADELPHIA, PA 19103-2899

Managing Editor *(Name and complete mailing address)*
PATRICK MANLEY, ELSEVIER INC.
1600 JOHN F KENNEDY BLVD. SUITE 1800
PHILADELPHIA, PA 19103-2899

10. Owner *(Do not leave blank. If the publication is owned by a corporation, give the name and address of the corporation immediately followed by the names and addresses of all stockholders owning or holding 1 percent or more of the total amount of stock. If not owned by a corporation, give the names and addresses of the individual owners. If owned by a partnership or other unincorporated firm, give its name and address as well as those of each individual owner. If the publication is published by a nonprofit organization, give its name and address.)*

Full Name	Complete Mailing Address
WHOLLY OWNED SUBSIDIARY OF REED/ELSEVIER, US HOLDINGS	1600 JOHN F KENNEDY BLVD. SUITE 1800 PHILADELPHIA, PA 19103-2899

11. Known Bondholders, Mortgagees, and Other Security Holders Owning or Holding 1 Percent or More of Total Amount of Bonds, Mortgages, or Other Securities. If none, check box. ▸ ☐ None

Full Name	Complete Mailing Address
N/A	

12. Tax Status *(For completion by nonprofit organizations authorized to mail at nonprofit rates)* *(Check one)*
The purpose, function, and nonprofit status of this organization and the exempt status for federal income tax purposes:
☒ Has Not Changed During Preceding 12 Months
☐ Has Changed During Preceding 12 Months *(Publisher must submit explanation of change with this statement)*

PS Form **3526**, July 2014 *(Page 1 of 4 (see instructions page 4))* PSN: 7530-01-000-9931 PRIVACY NOTICE: See our privacy policy on www.usps.com

---

13. Publication Title
EMERGENCY MEDICINE CLINICS OF NORTH AMERICA

14. Issue Date for Circulation Data Below
MAY 2022

15. Extent and Nature of Circulation

		Average No. Copies Each Issue During Preceding 12 Months	No. Copies of Single Issue Published Nearest to Filing Date
a. Total Number of Copies *(Net press run)*		250	219
b. Paid Circulation *(By Mail and Outside the Mail)*	(1) Mailed Outside-County Paid Subscriptions Stated on PS Form 3541 (include paid distribution above nominal rate, advertiser's proof copies, and exchange copies)	136	84
	(2) Mailed In-County Paid Subscriptions Stated on PS Form 3541 (include paid distribution above nominal rate, advertiser's proof copies, and exchange copies)	0	0
	(3) Paid Distribution Outside the Mails Including Sales Through Dealers and Carriers, Street Vendors, Counter Sales, and Other Paid Distribution Outside USPS®	58	53
	(4) Paid Distribution by Other Classes of Mail Through the USPS (e.g. First-Class Mail®)	0	0
c. Total Paid Distribution *(Sum of 15b (1), (2), (3), and (4))*	▸	194	137
d. Free or Nominal Rate Distribution *(By Mail and Outside the Mail)*	(1) Free or Nominal Rate Outside-County Copies included on PS Form 3541	39	65
	(2) Free or Nominal Rate In-County Copies Included on PS Form 3541	0	0
	(3) Free or Nominal Rate Copies Mailed at Other Classes Through the USPS (e.g. First-Class Mail)	0	0
	(4) Free or Nominal Rate Distribution Outside the Mail (Carriers or other means)	0	0
e. Total Free or Nominal Rate Distribution *(Sum of 15d (1), (2), (3) and (4))*	▸	39	65
f. Total Distribution *(Sum of 15c and 15e)*	▸	233	202
g. Copies not Distributed *(See Instructions to Publishers #4 (page #3))*	▸	17	17
h. Total *(Sum of 15f and g)*	▸	250	219
i. Percent Paid *(15c divided by 15f times 100)*		83.26%	67.82%

* If you are claiming electronic copies, go to line 16 on page 3. If you are not claiming electronic copies, skip to line 17 on page 3.

16. Electronic Copy Circulation

	Average No. Copies Each Issue During Preceding 12 Months	No. Copies of Single Issue Published Nearest to Filing Date
a. Paid Electronic Copies	▸	
b. Total Paid Print Copies (Line 15c) + Paid Electronic Copies (Line 16a)	▸	
c. Total Print Distribution (Line 15f) + Paid Electronic Copies (Line 16a)	▸	
d. Percent Paid (Both Print & Electronic Copies) (16b divided by 16c × 100)	▸	

☒ I certify that 50% of all my distributed copies (electronic and print) are paid above a nominal price.

17. Publication of Statement of Ownership
☒ If the publication is a general publication, publication of this statement is required. Will be printed in the NOVEMBER 2022 issue of this publication.
☐ Publication not required.

18. Signature and Title of Editor, Publisher, Business Manager, or Owner

Malathi Samayan - Distribution Controller

Malathi Samayan

Date 9/18/2022

I certify that all information furnished on this form is true and complete. I understand that anyone who furnishes false or misleading information on this form or who omits material or information requested on the form may be subject to criminal sanctions (including fines and imprisonment) and/or civil sanctions (including civil penalties).

PS Form **3526**, July 2014 *(Page 3 of 4)* PRIVACY NOTICE: See our privacy policy on www.usps.com

Moving?

Make sure your subscription moves with you!

To notify us of your new address, find your **Clinics Account Number** (located on your mailing label above your name), and contact customer service at:

Email: **journalscustomerservice-usa@elsevier.com**

800-654-2452 (subscribers in the U.S. & Canada)
314-447-8871 (subscribers outside of the U.S. & Canada)

Fax number: 314-447-8029

Elsevier Health Sciences Division
Subscription Customer Service
3251 Riverport Lane
Maryland Heights, MO 63043

*To ensure uninterrupted delivery of your subscription, please notify us at least 4 weeks in advance of move.

Printed and bound by CPI Group (UK) Ltd, Croydon, CR0 4YY

08/05/2025

01864723-0001